Multiple Factors in the Causation of Environmentally Induced Disease

ENVIRONMENTAL SCIENCES

An Interdisciplinary Monograph Series

EDITORS

DOUGLAS H. K. LEE
National Institute of
Environmental Health Sciences
Research Triangle Park
North Carolina

E. WENDELL HEWSON
Department of
Atmospheric Science
Oregon State University
Corvallis, Oregon

DANIEL OKUN
Department of Environmental
Sciences and Engineering
University of North Carolina
Chapel Hill, North Carolina

ARTHUR C. STERN, editor, AIR POLLUTION, Second Edition. In three volumes, 1968

L. FISHBEIN, W. G. FLAMM, and H. L. FALK, CHEMICAL MUTAGENS: Environmental Effects on Biological Systems, 1970

DOUGLAS H. K. LEE and DAVID MINARD, editors, PHYSIOLOGY, ENVIRONMENT, AND MAN, 1970

KARL D. KRYTER, THE EFFECTS OF NOISE ON MAN, 1970

R. E. MUNN, BIOMETEOROLOGICAL METHODS, 1970

M. M. KEY, L. E. KERR, and M. BUNDY, PULMONARY REACTIONS TO COAL DUST: "A Review of U. S. Experience," 1971

DOUGLAS H. K. LEE, editor, METALLIC CONTAMINANTS AND HUMAN HEALTH, 1972

DOUGLAS H. K. LEE, editor, ENVIRONMENTAL FACTORS IN RESPIRATORY DISEASE, 1972

H. ELDON SUTTON and MAUREEN I. HARRIS, editors, MUTAGENIC EFFECTS OF ENVIRONMENTAL CONTAMINANTS, 1972

RAY T. OGLESBY, CLARENCE A. CARLSON, and JAMES A. McCANN, editors, RIVER ECOLOGY AND MAN, 1972

LESTER V. CRALLEY, LEWIS T. CRALLEY, GEORGE D. CLAYTON, and JOHN A. JURGIEL, editors, INDUSTRIAL ENVIRONMENTAL HEALTH: The Worker and the Community, 1972

MOHAMED K. YOUSEF, STEVEN M. HORVATH, and ROBERT W. BULLARD, PHYSIOLOGICAL ADAPTATIONS: Desert and Mountain, 1972

DOUGLAS H. K. LEE and PAUL KOTIN, editors, MULTIPLE FACTORS IN THE CAUSATION OF ENVIRONMENTALLY INDUCED DISEASE, 1972

In preparation

MERRIL EISENBUD, ENVIRONMENTAL RADIOACTIVITY, Second Edition

ACADEMIC PRESS RAPID MANUSCRIPT REPRODUCTION

Fogarty International Center Proceedings No. 12

Multiple Factors in the Causation of Environmentally Induced Disease

Scientific Editors

Douglas H. K. Lee

NATIONAL INSTITUTE OF
ENVIRONMENTAL HEALTH SCIENCES
RESEARCH TRIANGLE PARK, NORTH CAROLINA

Paul Kotin

TEMPLE UNIVERSITY
PHILADELPHIA, PENNSYLVANIA

Sponsored by
National Institute of Environmental Health Sciences
Research Triangle Park, North Carolina
and
John E. Fogarty International Center
National Institutes of Health
Bethesda, Maryland

Academic Press
New York and London 1972

ACADEMIC PRESS, INC.
111 Fifth Avenue, New York, New York 10003

United Kingdom Edition published by
ACADEMIC PRESS, INC. (LONDON) LTD.
24/28 Oval Road,
London NW1 7DD

LIBRARY OF CONGRESS CATALOG CARD NUMBER: 72-82043

THE OPINIONS EXPRESSED IN THIS BOOK ARE THOSE OF THE
RESPECTIVE AUTHORS AND DO NOT NECESSARILY REPRESENT THOSE
OF THE DEPARTMENT OF HEALTH, EDUCATION, AND WELFARE.

PRINTED IN THE UNITED STATES OF AMERICA

CONTENTS

CHAPTER 1. INTRODUCTION: CONCEPTS OF MULTIPLE FACTORS
Brian MacMahon

PART 1. DISEASES OF MULTIFACTOR ORIGIN

CHAPTER 2. CANCER: A DISEASE INVOLVING MULTIPLE FACTORS
Paul Kotin

CHAPTER 3. POTENTIAL CONTRIBUTIONS OF MULTIPLE RISK FACTORS TO THE ETIOLOGY OF CIRRHOSIS
Thomas C. Chalmers

CHAPTER 4. MULTIPLE FACTOR ETIOLOGY IN CORONARY HEART DISEASE

Jerome Cornfield

CHAPTER 5. MULTIPLE FACTOR ETIOLOGY IN CHRONIC OBSTRUCTIVE LUNG DISEASE

Jerome Kleinerman

CHAPTER 6. MULTIPLE FACTORS IN THE CAUSATION OF RENAL DISEASE

Edward H. Kass

PART II. MECHANISMS OF MULTIFACTOR EFFECT

PART III. COMPLICATIONS INTRODUCED BY STORAGE OF CAUSATIVE AGENTS

CHAPTER 14. COMMENTS AND PERSPECTIVES
Douglas H. K. Lee

ORGANIZING PANEL

Frank R. Blood, * Director, Center for Toxicology, Vanderbilt University School of Medicine, Nashville, Tennessee 37203

Peter G. Condliffe, Chief, Conference and Seminar Program Branch, Fogarty International Center, National Institutes of Health, Bethesda, Maryland 20014

Paul Kotin, Vice President for Health Sciences, Temple University, Philadelphia, Pennsylvania 19140

Douglas H. K. Lee, Associate Director, National Institute of Environmental Health Sciences, Research Triangle Park, North Carolina 27709

James L. Whittenberger, Head, Department of Physiology, Harvard School of Public Health, Boston, Massachusetts 02115

* The untimely death of Dr. Blood before completion of this volume is much regretted.

CONTRIBUTORS

Lester Breslow, School of Public Health, University of California at Los Angeles, Los Angeles, California 90024

A. B. Brill, Vanderbilt University, Nashville, Tennessee 37203

Thomas C. Chalmers, Clinical Center, National Institutes of Health, Bethesda, Maryland 20014

Jerome Cornfield, Federation of American Societies of Experimental Biology, Bethesda, Maryland 20014

Kenneth P. Dubois, Toxicity Laboratory, University of Chicago, Chicago, Illinois 60637

James R. Fouts, National Institute of Environmental Health Sciences, Research Triangle Park, North Carolina 27709

G. W. Gibbs, Department of Epidemiology and Health, McGill University, Montreal, Canada

James R. Gillette, National Heart and Lung Institute, Bethesda, Maryland 20014

Wayland J. Hayes, Jr., Vanderbilt University School of Medicine, Nashville, Tennessee 37203

R. E. Johnston, Vanderbilt University, Nashville, Tennessee 37203

Edward H. Kass, Channing Laboratory, Thorndike Memorial Laboratory, Harvard Medical School, and Boston City Hospital, Boston, Massachusetts 02115

Jerome Kleinerman, Department of Pathology, St. Luke's Hospital, and Case Western Reserve University School of Medicine, Cleveland, Ohio 44104

Paul Kotin, Temple University, Philadelphia, Pennsylvania 19140

Douglas H. K. Lee, National Institute of Environmental Health Sciences, Research Triangle Park, North Carolina 27709

Brian MacMahon, Department of Epidemiology, Harvard School of Public Health, Boston, Massachusetts 02115

J. C. McDonald, Department of Epidemiology and Health, McGill University, Montreal, Canada

J. Manfreda, Department of Epidemiology and Health, McGill University, Montreal, Canada

Jerry Mitchell, National Heart and Lung Institute, Bethesda, Maryland 20014

Robert A. Neal, Vanderbilt University School of Medicine, Nashville, Tennessee 37203

F. L. Parker, Vanderbilt University, Nashville, Tennessee 37203

Harold Sandstead, Vanderbilt University School of Medicine, Nashville, Tennessee 37203

F. M. M. White, Department of Epidemiology and Health, McGill University, Montreal, Canada

EDITORIAL COMMENT

As governmental and public interest in environmental quality increases, and as conservation or remedial programs are planned, a number of scientists are called upon for advice or decision in areas involving fields beyond their own personal expertise. Program managers, experienced in administration, also find themselves in need of information on technical matters that fall within their jurisdiction.

The announcement that a United Nations Conference on human environment was to be held in Stockholm in June 1972 pointed out the fact that these needs are worldwide. It stimulated the John E. Fogarty International Center of the National Institutes of Health to investigate how these needs might be met. In conjunction with the National Institute of Environmental Health Sciences, also part of the National Institutes of Health, a decision was made to prepare four books on the aspects of environmental health for which suitable résumés were not readily available.

The interplay of multiple factors in the causation of environmentally related disease was the topic selected for the fourth of the set. As for the other volumes, a small panel of experts in the field was asked to delimit the scope that should be followed, to indicate the specific topics within that scope, and to suggest other experts who could contribute to the volume. Contributors brought draft papers to a three-day workshop where the drafts were thoroughly discussed, amendments suggested, and integration among chapters developed. Extensive editing followed.

The contributors to the previous three books had a relatively easy task in that they were asked to condense existing knowledge on the particular subjects into a form that would be instructive for scientists and scientific managers who had to make decisions involving fields in which they were not themselves expert. The contributors for this fourth book had a much more difficult task. They were, in effect, asked to comment in learned fashion on a concept rather than on factual information. The concept, moreover, was one which is often invoked but seldom defined. The previous three books, in presenting relatively hard knowledge, revealed their own areas of deficiency, such as lack of information on the environmental distribution of stressors or the poor comparability of information on even closely related stressors. This book goes further in repeatedly revealing that the information necessary for good comprehension and sound recommendation is simply not readily at hand. It is believed, however, that the very demonstration of deficiencies is important, and that the development of a more adequate approach to environmental problems will result from attention being drawn to them.

After an introduction based mainly on the epidemiology of infectious disease, but applicable to other environmental factors, some diseases believed to have multiple etiological factors are reviewed in Part I. Part II goes to to the other end of the pathological spectrum and looks at disturbances of cellular processes resulting from two or more factors operating simultaneously or in succession. Part III examines the further complicating role that storage of potentially toxic material in body tissues and its subsequent release introduce into an already complex situation. Part IV deals with some implications of multiple factor operation.

It has not been easy to preserve a balance between simplification for the nonspecialist and adequacy as viewed by the expert. The text now appearing has been checked by the contributors, but we must accept responsibility for any undue selectivity that may have occurred as well as for errors of omission or commission. We hope, however, that the text will help those who need to know the state of current knowledge on the health significance of multiple environmental factors but who do not have the time to pursue the detailed literature or to seek a compilation directed to their special needs.

Douglas H. K. Lee
Paul Kotin

CONCENTRATION UNITS AND CONVERSION FACTORS

Metric and proportional units are used somewhat indiscriminately for indicating the concentration of toxic agents. In this volume the units preferred by the individual contributor have been retained. The reader who wishes to make comparisons between concentrations expressed in different units will find the following data useful.

In solid and liquid mixtures, proportional units refer to weights and are easily converted to metric equivalents:

$$1 \text{ part per million (ppm)} = 1 \text{ mg/kg}$$
$$1 \text{ part per billion (ppb)} = 1 \text{ } \mu\text{g/kg}$$
$$(1 \text{ kg of liquid of density } 1 = 1 \text{ li})$$

In gaseous mixtures, however, proportional units refer to volumes, so that conversion varies with the molecular weight of the dispersed substance, temperature, and barometric pressure. The conversion formula is

1 part per million by volume
at 25°C and 760 mm HG pressure = 0.041 (molecular weight) mg/m^3

Note: The factor 0.041 represents $273/(298 \times 22.4)$

Particulate matter in air is often expressed in terms of millions of particles per cubic foot or per cubic meter. To convert from cubic foot to cubic meter, multiply by 35.3. (This also gives particles per cubic centimeter.)

Multiple Factors
in the
Causation of
Environmentally
Induced Disease

CHAPTER 1. INTRODUCTION:
CONCEPTS OF MULTIPLE FACTORS

BRIAN MACMAHON, Department of Epidemiology, Harvard School of Public Health, Boston, Massachusetts

Almost 2400 years ago, Hippocrates pointed out the need to understand the causes of disease if we are to control it. Only in the last one hundred years, however, have we begun to make measurable progress in this direction. In this brief span of time many living and inanimate agents capable of inducing human disease have been identified. The reductions in mortality and morbidity that have followed are clear -- at least in those areas of the world fortunate enough to possess the resources to apply the knowledge for the benefit of their populations.

For many years after the beginning of this era of discovery the guiding philosophy was that each human ailment had its own particular cause, in much the same way that each force had its own equal and opposite reaction. This philosophy was most vividly expressed in the postulates of Koch -- a set of "rules" that for many decades specified the conditions that must be met if a particular microbe was to be considered the cause of a particular human illness. The concept, in general, served us well, providing the means for controlling many infectious and chemically-induced diseases.

As the list of factors known to be capable of inducing human disease has lengthened, it has become clear that a particular disease manifestation may have more than one causal antecedent. In addition we have learned that exposure to a known cause of illness does not always lead to the expression of that illness and that identification of a causal antecedent does not necessarily provide the ability

1

to prevent or control the ailment. We have come to recognize that the one cause-one disease model is too simple. Illness in an individual is the result of a multitude of prior circumstances -- including those multiple, independent, minor circumstances that we call chance -- and causal circumstances differ from one individual to another, even when the manifestations of their illness are indistinguishable. Seemingly minor differences in diet or in physical or chemical environment determine the reaction of a person to a given microbial or genetic stimulus, and vice versa. Indeed the causal antecedents of illness in any individual comprise a web of intertwined circumstances that in their full breadth and complexity lie quite beyond our understanding.

PRACTICAL UTILITY OF THE CONCEPT OF MULTIPLE FACTOR ETIOLOGY

It may appear that, in our recognition of the complexity of disease etiology, we have gone from one extreme to the other -- from the limited utility of the one cause-one disease model to a philosophy that, because of the limitations of our ability to comprehend, may be of no more, and perhaps even less, practical utility for the development of disease control measures. Fortunately, to develop effective control measures it is not necessary to understand the entire causal web but merely to identify significant strands, the disruption of which can lead to alteration in the whole structure. Recognition of the possibility of multiple etiology -- even when we know that we can never understand the antecedents of a particular illness in their entirety -- enormously increases the opportunities for preventive action since it increases the number of points at which such action can be effected. This is clearly illustrated by two kinds of situation:

1. A factor is identified as an unequivocal cause of disease but proves to be not manipulatable for preventive purposes. Genes generally fall into this class. It may then be possible to identify other components of the causal web that can be altered. Phenylketonuria, for example, is a disease that thirty years ago

2

might have been considered a single factor disease -- determined exclusively by the presence of a single recessive gene in homozygous form. Certainly it appeared that everybody carrying the required genetic combination manifested the disease. The discovery that the manifestation depended, in addition, on the presence of phenylalanine in the diet opened the way for the prevention of at least some of the disease manifestations.

2. A factor that causes disease also has desirable effects that make its elimination unacceptable, or at least less acceptable than other ways of achieving the health objective. For example, the community at large appears to find unacceptable the elimination of cigarettes as a measure to prevent the more than 100,000 deaths that these cause annually. In spite of the availability of measures directed against specific microbial causes of enteric diseases, prevention of such diseases in this country is still based on the provision of unadulterated water and food rather than on what would have to be massive vaccination programs.

The concept of multiple-factor etiology often appears to be used as a last refuge by investigators unable to identify any causal factor of significance. As such the term has a pessimistic ring. We should recognize, therefore, that the existence of multiple etiologic factors provides us more, rather than less, opportunities for preventive action.

THE CHANGING CAUSES OF DISEASE

The profile of the human environment -- and for that matter of the human gene pool -- is in a constant state of flux. The microbial and other living agents of a disease to which a typical North American is now exposed are considerably less varied and less widely distributed than those of fifty years ago. Also more homogeneous is the general ecological milieu that hosts such agents. On the other hand, exposures to physical and chemical substances -- of which some are known to cause disease and many are suspected of doing so -- is increasing astronomically. The gene pool is changing as the result of the breakdown (and formation) of breeding isolates, and of changes in frequency of inter-ethnic matings and consanguinity -- not to mention the consequences of our own interference in the selective processes that have played such a large part in the moulding of our present genetic inheritance.

Moreover, the social environment is undergoing rapid modification, leading to revision of priorities in the attack on disease and to changes in the points at which, and methods whereby, attempts are made to control disease processes.

Here we have yet another consideration that makes the concept of multiple-factor etiology important. If we are aware and knowledgeable of the many antecedents of illness, we extend our opportunities for preventive and control measures so that the specific measure or measures used best fit the needs and wishes of the population of the time, and can be modified as the milieu changes.

ACUTE AND CHRONIC DISEASE

The thought is frequently expressed that the etiology of the chronic diseases is more complex than that of the acute infections or toxic reactions, for which at least some causal factors have already been identified, and that the concept of multiple-factor etiology is somehow more relevant to the former than the latter. This belief seems to arise from several sources:

1. Problems always appear to be more complicated before they have been solved than after.

2. There are examples of causal factors -- notably some forms of acute infection (such as vaccinia) and certain toxic agents -- that will produce illness in virtually every individual in an exposed population.

4

3. In some acute diseases -- again notably those due to certain infections or toxic agents -- there is a close correspondence between the group of patients classified together by virtue of being exposed to a specific causal agent and the group classified in terms of manifestational criteria. Diseases due to measles or rabies virus would be examples.

4. There are infectious diseases -- poliomyelitis, for example -- in which there is clear evidence of multiple etiology but which nevertheless have been, or could be, controlled by attention to a single etiologic agent.

None of these considerations reduces the importance of multiple factors in the etiology of the acute infectious diseases, and all apply with equal force to the degenerative diseases, chronic intoxications and other chronic diseases as to the acute infections. All disease manifestations have multiple causes. What is usually at issue is not how many factors are involved in the production of a particular disease, but how many we need to know about to prevent or control it most effectively. The roles of tonsillectomy and heavy exercise in the etiology of poliomyelitis were of substantially greater interest before the development of a control measure based on another causal factor, the virus, than they are at the present time. Knowledge of the role of cigarette smoking in the lung cancer of uranium miners derives considerable importance from the practical difficulties that are involved in the prevention of the disease by measures directed towards the radiation exposure alone.

DIFFERENT CONCEPTS OF MULTIPLE-FACTOR ETIOLOGY

Although much has been said and written about multiple-factor etiology, rarely is the meaning of the term defined. There are, conceptually, at least three different sets of circumstances that are implied:

1. Several factors may be necessary for the induction of a mechanism that finally leads to disease manifestations. For example, a

particular type of cell may have to be in a particular physiologic state before contact with a microbiologic agent will initiate an invasive process. The place and time of occurrence may not be the same for all the factors involved. Thus, changes in a cell induced by viral infection in infancy may not demonstrate malignancy until the appearance of a particular hormonal environment many years later. Tuberculosis may not be established in lung cells until they are damaged by the action of silica dust. Nevertheless, the concept is of a multiplicity of factors forming a single constellation of causes which results in the induction of a particular disease manifestation.

2. A second concept often implied is that each of the individual factors in such a basic constellation has its own constellation of determinants, so that any one of them can be altered -- and the basic constellation therefore changed -- through a variety of mechanisms. One may enclose milling machinery, have operators wear masks, or substitute glass fibers for asbestos -- all will reduce the risk of asbestos fibers producing lung disease.

3. A third concept is that identical disease manifestations -- or at least manifestations that cannot be distinguished on the basis of present knowledge -- may be associated with quite different basic constellations of etiologic factors. For example, in mice, cleft palate can be induced by inbreeding, anoxia, vitamin deficiency, or a variety of chemical or physical exposures. Whether there is some final common pathway that can be triggered by any one of these various agents is a moot question. One may believe that specific effects are always produced by specific constellations of causes, and that apparent exceptions to this principle result only from our inability to identify final common pathways, to lack of specificity in the definition of causal factors, or to our

failure to distinguish manifestations that are in fact different. If so, this category of multiple causality is identical with the first. However, there are certainly many situations -- in man as well as in animals -- in which for practical purposes we must act on the supposition that identical manifestations may result from different constellations of causes.

SYNERGY IN MULTIPLE-FACTOR ETIOLOGY

The situation with respect to phenylketonuria described above is a relatively simple one. The disease appears to depend on the completion of both of only two independent processes, blockage of either one of which results in the absence of disease. Dose-response relationships appear not to be of appreciable significance. More frequently, in those situations involving more than one cause that have been investigated in man -- and they are quite few in number -- we are faced not with a present-or-absent situation, but with continuous variation in the frequency of disease associated with variation in the strength, as well as the number, of factors involved.

Suppose, for example, that we are dealing with two factors, both of which are associated with the same disease. Usually, there is some "background" level of the disease that is present in the absence of exposure to either factor, persons exposed to both factors have the highest risk, and persons exposed to only one of the factors have intermediate rates. An interesting and potentially useful exercise is then to determine whether persons exposed to both factors have more disease than would be expected if the two factors were operating independently of each other -- in other words, whether it appears that they are acting synergistically. Two examples will be given -- one of a situation in which there appears not to be a synergistic effect of the two factors, and one in which there does. However, there have been very few investigations of this type and the conclusions from the two sets of data to be presented have not been confirmed. They are presented only to illustrate the principles involved.

7

Table 1 shows data on occupational exposure and cigarette smoking in cases and controls in a study of bladder cancer in Eastern Massachusetts conducted by Cole and others (1,2). From the usual formula used in case-control studies, one can compute, from the numbers of cases and controls, the series of relative risks shown in the fifth column of the table. These express the risk in each exposure category relative to an arbitrarily assigned risk of 1.00 for men with neither exposure. Using these relative risks, and assuming that the distribution of the population with respect to exposure is similar to that of the controls, one can estimate (3) the annual rates in each of the four exposure categories that would be necessary to produce the overall bladder cancer rate of 41.8 per 100,000 observed in this population. These are given in the next column of the table. We see that men exposed to either one of the factors have rates higher than those exposed to neither (as reflected also in the relative risks of 2.00 and 2.84). We can, furthermore, compute the amount of each rate that can be attributed to each exposure, on the assumption that the higher rate is indeed attributable to the exposure and not the result of some unidentified non-causal association. The amount of the rate among smokers that is "attributable" to smoking then is 40.6 minus 20.3, or 20.3 per 100,000. Similarly, the attributable risk among those occupationally exposed who were non-smokers is 57.7 minus 20.3, or 37.4 per 100,000.

If the two factors, occupational exposure and cigarette smoking, were operating independently one might expect the attributable risk for persons exposed to both to be approximately the sum of the two attributable risks (less some very small correction to compensate for the problem of competing risks). The observed attributable risk for those exposed to both factors, 48 per 100,000, is indeed quite similar to the sum of the independent risks, 58 per 100,000, suggesting that the two factors are acting independently and are not associated with higher rates when they act in concert than when they act independently.

It is sometimes desirable to evaluate the additivity of risks when actual rates are not known. If the relative risks in the various exposure categories are known, a value which can be treated in

TABLE 1 -- BLADDER CANCER IN EASTERN MASSACHUSETTS, ACCORDING TO EXPOSURE TO
OCCUPATIONAL RISK AND/OR CIGARETTE SMOKING. MALES, 20-89 YEARS OF AGE.

High risk occupation[1]	Cigarette smoking[2]	Number of Cases	Number of Controls	Relative risk (R)	Estimated annual rate per 100,000	Attributable annual rate per 100,000	R-1
No	No	43	94	1.00	20.3	0.0	0.00
No	Yes	173	189	2.00	40.6	20.3	1.00
Yes	No	26	20	2.84	57.7	37.4	1.84
Yes	Yes	111	72	3.37	68.4	48.1	2.37
Total		353	375	-	41.8	-	-

[1] "Yes" = has ever worked in an industry shown in this study to be associated with increased risk

[2] "Yes" = has smoked at least 100 cigarettes in his life.

Data provided by Dr. Philip Cole

a fashion similar to that of attributable rates is obtained by subtracting 1.0 from each of the relative risks (4). These values are shown in the last column of Table 1. Thus, in this instance, the ratio of the sums of the independent excess risks to the risk manifested by the group with both exposures is the same if it is computed on the figures in the final column (2.84:2.37) as if it is computed on the actual attributable rates (57.5:48.1).

This procedure is necessary in the next example, given in Table 2, of an apparently synergistic effect of blood type and oral contraceptive use in the production of venous thromboembolism. Jick et al. (5) have shown that risk of thromboembolism is higher among persons of blood types other than 0 than among those of blood type 0, and that the relative risk associated with blood type is higher among users than among non-users of oral contraceptives. These authors do not give relative risks associated with oral contraceptive use, but such data have been provided by Sartwell et al. (6). Using the data from these two studies, the estimates shown in Table 2 have been derived. In this instance the excess risk experienced by persons exposed to both risk factors (7.4) far exceeds the sum of the excess risks associated with each single exposure (2.3). It appears that cigarette smoking and asbestos exposure, and cigarette smoking and uranium mining, also act in this synergistic fashion to cause lung cancer, but in neither situation are available data sufficient to yield quantitative comparisons of the risks associated with the independent exposures and that experienced by persons with combined exposures.

What conclusions can be drawn from the presence or absence of synergism between different etiologic factors? It is tempting to suppose that simple additivity of excess risks implies that the different factors belong to different constellations of causes of the disease. That is, that they are indicative of the type of multiple causality in which different constellations of causes are producing manifestations that, if not identical, are at least not distinguishable on the basis of current knowledge. Synergism, on the other hand, may suggest that the different factors are part of the same constellation of causes that is responsible for a common single

TABLE 2 -- ESTIMATED DISTRIBUTION OF A SET OF THEORETICAL
CASES OF THROMBOEMBOLISM AND CONTROLS BY ORAL
CONTRACEPTIVE USE AND BLOOD TYPE.

Use of oral contraceptive	Blood type	Percent of Cases	Percent of Controls	Relative risk (R)	R-1
No	0	21	41	1.0	0.0
No	Not 0	41	46	1.7	0.7
Yes	0	8	6	2.6	1.6
Yes	Not 0	30	7	8.4	7.4
Total	Total	100	100	-	-

The distributions are estimated from the data of Jick
et al. (5) (USA only) and Sartwell et al. (6). The
theoretical distributions of cases and controls are based
on data in the two studies whenever possible, and otherwise
are estimated as being such as to give the relative risks
reported in the two studies.

final mechanism for the induction of the
manifestations. This implication stems from the
logarithmic form of many dose-response curves, and
the supposition that the two independent factors may
either be acting as a single factor or that one of
the factors increases the availability of the other
-- in each case prompting a logarithmic increase in
response to an arithmetic increase in dose.

However, we have as yet insufficient information
to draw any firm conclusions about the meaning of
various forms of interaction between factors. There
are still few diseases for which more than one
specific cause is known, and even fewer for which
quantitative estimates of risk associated with each
cause -- alone and in combination -- can be made.
Only when we have very markedly expanded this list
will we be able to categorize the kinds of
interaction that are observed and relate them
empirically to known types of disease-producing
mechanisms. It should be noted, however, that even
if a particular synergism cannot be interpreted
explicitly in terms of mechanism, the knowledge may
still be put to practical use -- as, for example, in
the case of cigarette smoking and uranium mining.

Both from practical and from conceptual points of view, therefore, the continued exploration of interaction effects in quantitative terms is an important area for investigation.

REFERENCES

1. Cole, P. et al. (1971). Smoking and cancer of the lower urinary tract. New Eng. J. Med. 284: 129.

2. Cole, P. et al. (1972). Occupation and cancer of the lower urinary tract. Cancer 29: 1250.

3. MacMahon, B. and Pugh, T. F. (1971). Epidemiology. Principles and Methods. Little, Brown, Boston.

4. Cole, P. and MacMahon, B. (1971). Attributable risk percent in case-control studies. Brit. J. Prev. Soc. Med. 25: 242.

5. Jick, H. et al. (1969). Venous thromboembolic disease and ABO blood type. Lancet 1: 539.

6. Sartwell, P. et al. (1969). Thromboembolism and oral contraceptives: An epidemiologic case-control study. Amer. J. Epidemiol. 90: 365.

PART I

DISEASES OF MULTIFACTOR ORIGIN

In this Part contributors were asked to take certain well-known disease states and discuss the evidence for the operation of multiple environmental factors in the causation or development of the condition, with sufficient background on the disease state itself to put their operation in perspective.

CHAPTER 2. CANCER:
A DISEASE INVOLVING MULTIPLE FACTORS

PAUL KOTIN, Temple University,
Philadelphia, Pennsylvania

The categorical designation -- cancer -- encompasses a group of diseases caused by multiple factors acting singly or in combination. These factors are operative both in the external environment and in the host. Analytical studies in the environment, experimental studies in laboratory models, and clinical studies in man indicate with increasing certainty that a wide variety of chemicals and biological carcinogens may be causally related to cancers of specific tissues and organs. Carcinogens may act in an additive, synergistic or inhibitory manner, and differences in risk to cancer reported in populations reflect primarily environmental experiences and secondarily variations in genetic susceptibility. Age, sex, and physiologic state of the target tissues also modify cancer incidence. Where concordances between environmental, experimental, and clinical data are greatest, interactive causes have been clearly demonstrated. Where the environmental and experimental data are firm but data in man are less solid, the multifactorial aspect of etiology is still valid and may be applied to public health measures.

In the study of the natural history of cancer in man it is possible to describe a continuum which emphasizes its multifactorial etiology. The continuum is double stranded; one strand concerned with exogenous or environmental factors and the other with endogenous or host factors.

ENVIRONMENTAL CARCINOGENESIS

Environmental carcinogenesis is concerned with the identification of carcinogenic hazards, the elucidation of their mode of entry and mechanism of action in the host, and the characterization of populations affected by them. Variations in the occurrence of cancer in man have been identified in the past on the bases of occupation, site of residence, socio-economic or cultural characteristics or special ethnic considerations. Agents responsible for increased risks have been investigated by laboratory procedures directed to pinpointing specific causative factors in complex environments. Laboratory investigations of potential carcinogenic agents also have followed carcinogenic suspicion on the basis of the chemical structure of certain compounds either naturally present or artificially introduced into the environment.

Carcinogenicity from an experimental viewpoint is demonstrated by bioassay experiments in which the suspected agents are administered to test animals by feeding, subcutaneous or parenteral injection, skin painting or total body exposure in appropriately designed chambers. The disciplines applied in studying environmental carcinogenesis, therefore, consist of: (1) epidemiology with its allied sciences of biometry and statistics; (2) chemistry, both organic and synthetic, for the identification, purification, and laboratory preparation of known and suspected carcinogenic agents; (3) biochemistry, aimed at elucidating the anatomic and metabolic fate of carcinogenic agents; (4) experimental pathology, concerned with evaluating the response of biological systems from single cells, to intact hosts, to carcinogenic stimuli; and (5) virology, aimed at identifying viruses with oncogenic potential and studying their infectivity and the immune response to these agents.

During the past 50 years, there have been two general approaches to the study of cancer: basic laboratory investigation and field research. The former has been concerned with the study of the cell and of subcellular fractions down to the molecule itself, directed to the question, "Why and how do cells become cancerized?" Field research, on the other hand, with its somewhat differently oriented approach, seeks to answer the questions, "Why do people get cancer?" and "What is responsible for differences in susceptibility and resistance to cancer?" Each complements the other.

EXOGENOUS FACTORS

Environmental influences offer the most logical and acceptable explanation for the varied pattern of cancer occurrence. Chemicals producing cancer in a variety of anatomical sites have been identified in the environment of high risk groups. For some, the etiological relationships are clear; for example: aromatic amines and urinary bladder cancer, asbestos and mesothelioma, polycyclic aromatic hydrocarbons and skin cancer. For other sites, carcinogenic agents have as yet not been identified or their causal role not firmly established. Conversely, numerous carcinogenic agents have been identified in the environment where unusual risks to cancer have not been shown. It is, therefore, important to emphasize that the demonstration of a carcinogen in the environment need not inevitably connote a biological effect. The variety of stimuli that can cause cancer is shown in Table 1.

Following identification of carcinogens in the environment, there is a need to demonstrate biological availability -- the ability to gain host entry, reach target organs, and interact with cellular components concerned with the initiation of malignant transformation. The role of environmental factors in the induction of cancer can be evaluated in light of current concepts of the carcinogenic process.

It is known that a long period of time usually elapses between the time of onset of exposure to a carcinogen and the ultimate development of an overt cancer. As shown in Table 2, this latent period can be as little as a few years, or it can comprise a major segment of the total life span. The equivalent of this epidemiological observation can be remarkably duplicated in experimental models. It is during the latent period that environmental influences affecting cancer rates in diverse populations appear to primarily operate.

TABLE 1 -- CARCINOGENIC STIMULI

Chemical Carcinogens

Polycyclic Aromatic Hydrocarbons
benzo(a)pyrene
3-methylcholanthrene
dibenz(a,h)anthracene

Aromatic Amines and Amides
2-napthylamine
benzidine
4-aminobiphenyl
2-acetylaminofluorene
4-aminostilbene

Alkylating Agents
N-mustards
epoxides

Aminoazo Dyes
2',3-dimethyl-4-aminoazobenzene
4-dimethylaminoazobenzene

Miscellaneous Compounds
nitrosoamines
ethionine
thioacetamide
urethan
carbon tetrachloride
senecio alkaloids
aflatoxin
tannic acid
selenium

Hormones

Viruses
DNA Type
RNA Type

Radiation
Ionizing
Ultra-violet

Films
Plastic, metal, glass

TABLE 2 -- LATENT PERIODS OF OCCUPATIONAL CANCERS

Organ and Agent	Average Latent Period Years	Range of Latent Period Years
Skin		
Tar	20-24	1-50
Creosote Oil	25	15-40
Mineral Oil	50-54	4-75
Crude paraffin oil	15-18	3-35
Solar radiation	20-30	15-40
X-radiation	7	1-12
Lung		
Asbestos	18	15-21
Chromates	15	5-47
Nickel	22	6-30
Tar fumes	16	9-23
Ionizing radiation	25-35	7-50
Bladder		
Aromatic amines	11-15	2-40

There are three possible sequelae following initial interaction between the carcinogen and the cell: (1) the cell may die; (2) cancer will ultimately develop; or (3) exposure may be at a level insufficient to produce cancer within the normal life expectancy, unless the effect of other factors which may or may not be carcinogenic intervenes. With skin cancer as a model, it has been demonstrated that the development of cancer occurs in stages as outlined in Table 3. The stage of initiation is of short duration, irreversible, and specific. Chemicals producing this effect are identified as carcinogens. This is followed by the promotion or second stage of carcinogenesis which, in contrast, is of long duration, reversible, and capable of production by a wide variety of nonspecific chemical and physical influences. These agents are variously referred to

TABLE 3 -- TWO-STAGE MECHANISM OF CARCINOGENESIS

Initiation

1. Rapid
2. Specific
3. Irreversible
   a. Carcinogen

Promotion

1. Slow
2. Non-specific
3. Reversible
   a. Carcinogen
   b. Co-carcinogen   )
   c. Promoting agent   } synonyms
   d. Accelerator   )

as co-carcinogens, accelerators, or promoters. The modifying effect of environmental changes would seem to be greatest during the interval when co-carcinogenic factors are at play, but no stage in the origin and the development of cancer appears immune to the effect of multiple factors.

In summary, by definition, a carcinogen alone at an appropriate dose level can act as both an initiator and a promoter and produce cancer at any site during the normal life span. At the subthreshold or non-cancer producing level, the carcinogen acts only as an initiator and requires the help of co-carcinogens for the induction of cancer. In laboratory models, tumor yield is predictable when appropriate dose levels of carcinogens are administered. Alternatively, at a subthreshold dose, the ultimate cancer development is predictable with less certainty. While this sequence can be observed and elegantly quantified in highly inbred laboratory animal strains, it is subject to modification by a variety of host or endogenous influences under ordinary circumstances. Host factors operate by different mechanisms and pathways and have, I believe, clear though secondary relevance to the changing cancer patterns in populations.

The matter of biological availability is crucial. An arrow resting in the quiver is an innocuous environmental agent; shot from a bow it can become a lethal one. The release of the bow string has facilitated biological availability. As shown in Table 4, factors affecting this parameter segregate themselves into two components: those operative at the portal of entry and those related to the target

TABLE 4 -- FACTORS AFFECTING BIOLOGICAL AVAILABILITY OF CHEMICAL CARCINOGENS

(Portal of Entry)

1. Stability (environment)
2. Physical state (environment, host)
3. Solubility (environment, host)
4. Antecedent or concurrent disease (host)
5. Competency of physiologic defense mechanisms (host)

(Target Site)

1. Morphologic state of tissue(s)
2. Metabolic state of detoxification site(s)
3. Hormonal state

TABLE 5 -- SITES OF ACTION OF CHEMICAL CARCINOGENS

1. Portal of entry; e.g., skin cancers from polynuclear aromatic hydrocarbons
2. Site of elective localization; e.g., bone cancer from radium, leukemia from benzene
3. Site of detoxification; e.g., liver cancer from azo dyes or aflatoxin
4. Site of excretion; e.g., urinary bladder cancer from aromatic amines.

site. In consequence, carcinogens may act at one or more of several sites (Table 5).

The respiratory tract provides an example of portal of entry effect. In the respiratory tract particle size is critical; there is a finite size range for lung penetration; and, within the lung, size also determines site of deposition. Carcinogens also vary in their chemical properties, and this too can determine their ability to overcome host defenses and initiate disease. Respiratory carcinogens are found in several environmental sites (work place, polluted air, cigarette smoke); all are chemically complex, and irritants interfering with the normal flow of the mucous blanket on the respiratory epithelium usually accompany the carcinogen. The effect of these irritants and their ability to promote abnormal retention of particles enhance cell-carcinogen contact, thereby facilitating interaction. The consequence of the combined repetitive inhalation of carcinogens and chemicals neutralizing the mucociliary defenses is entirely compatible with the first steps on the induction of lung cancer.

ENDOGENOUS FACTORS

The metabolic state of an appropriate anatomic site can effectively serve to portray the role of host factors. The metabolic handling of carcinogens may be looked upon as a second line of defense if we consider the mechanical barriers of epithelia as the first. Carcinogenic chemicals undergo metabolic change in a manner similar to that of drugs. For the most part, metabolic alteration of environmental agents in the host results in detoxification. In carcinogenesis there are several notorious examples where the reverse is true. Often an agent in its environmental state may not be carcinogenic and only become so after metabolic alteration. Although the metabolism of carcinogens is an endogenous event, the biochemical mechanisms are sensitive to environmental influences. Enzymes involved in the metabolic conversion of chemical carcinogens primarily belong to a group called induced enzymes; i.e., they are synthesized in the cell in response to the stimulation resulting from the entry of the carcinogen into the cell. Individuals may vary in their ability to synthesize these enzymes. This ability is to a significant degree affected by the other factors listed in Table 6. Age of onset of exposure is an important determinant. Recent research has established the increased susceptibility of the newborn of mammalian species to the action of a carcinogen. There are several examples of compounds which showed uncertain carcinogenicity when bioassayed exclusively in adults, but which were potent inducers of tumors when tested in the newborn. The exquisite susceptibility of the newborn to chemical carcinogenesis may well be the result of failure to respond to the enzyme-inducing effect of the carcinogen.

22

TABLE 6 -- FACTORS MODIFYING HOST RESPONSE

1. Age
2. Sex
3. Nutrition
4. Physiologic state of metabolic sites
5. Congenital abnormalities
6. Antecedent or concurrent disease

The physiological state of the organism is also a factor governing the efficiency of enzyme synthesis. When to this is added the increased susceptibility that may be inherent in the abnormal cells of diseased organs, independent of causation, the development of high-risk or preneoplastic states becomes understandable; e.g.: cirrhosis in relation to cancer of the liver; hyperplasia to cancer of the endocrine glands; ulcerative colitis to cancer of the colon; and intestinalization of stomach mucosa to cancer of the stomach. Interference with detoxification mechanisms, even at subtle levels for short periods of time, can result in the persistence and enhanced action of the carcinogen.

While differences in cancer incidence in the male and female are most obvious for genital and accessory genital organs, significant differences exist for cancer of visceral organs as well. These differences suggest hormonal influences at work, and indeed data indicate that they are operative in many ways. The rates and patterns of induction of enzymes differ in the male and female. Hormonal differences may indirectly modify the action of chemical carcinogens by their effect on cell membrane permeability. Estrogenic and androgenic hormones significantly modify the entry of particulate matter into cells in experimental models. There is evidence that the same applies to man, and this suggests itself as one of the bases for the variation in cancer rates for certain sites during the three periods of contrasting hormonal activity: pre-puberty, sexual maturity, and the climacteric.

COMMENT

The traditional division of environmental carcinogenic agents into chemical, physical, and viral carcinogens on the basis of their properties has, until very recently, suffered from the assumption that each group was a domain unto itself, acting to a greater or lesser degree independently of the other two. A significant recent development in cancer research has been the recognition that individual carcinogenic agents of these different classes may act in combination or, as some recent data indicate, the effect of one may be mediated through the other. Neoplasms can be induced predictably in a wide variety of mammalian species using agents of any of the three classes. The term "carcinogen" incidentally is generic, as tumors can be induced in tissues derived from all three germ layers, so that sarcomas as well as carcinomas can result.

Man was the first species in which chemical carcinogenesis was demonstrated -- scrotal cancer in chimney sweeps. Later systematic studies have necessarily involved animal experiments, and a critical question relating to all laboratory investigations in chemical carcinogenesis concerns their applicability to man. Certain limitations are inherent in data derived from laboratory studies. There are distinct differences between the circumstances of exposure in the laboratory and the human situation. Experiments under controlled conditions using pure chemical reagents, defined animal species and strains, and elegant techniques are necessary for the elucidation of the mechanisms of carcinogenesis. Despite the limitations resulting from these artifactitious circumstances, chemical agents proven to be carcinogenic by bioassay, utilizing any of the several modes of administration in one or more experimental species, should be regarded as hazardous, and elimination, if possible, or rigid control in the environment should be undertaken. However, since a carcinogen-free environment is a virtual impossibility and potent carcinogens are almost self-identifying, it becomes imperative to investigate the effect of suspect chemicals, including weak carcinogens, in relation to the total exposure of man. This offers the dual benefit of placing experimentally proven carcinogens in perspective and perhaps of identifying agents heretofore erroneously assumed to be free of carcinogenic hazards. Further weak carcinogens are especially likely to participate in a multifactorial constellation.

DEFINITION OF CURRENT BOUNDARY BETWEEN KNOWLEDGE AND IGNORANCE

Traditionally, epidemiological data identifying unusual carcinogenic risks have served as the basis for laboratory studies aimed at dissecting various factors in the high risk environment, with the hope of ultimately singling out the responsible agent or agents. Of equal significance, though essentially neglected until now, is the need to utilize existing laboratory data in the interpretation of epidemiological findings. It is imperative that the observations of cancer in man be evaluated in the light of accumulated knowledge in experimental carcinogenesis. The significance of experimentally weak carcinogens is barely, if at all, understood. The role of cigarette smoking in the pathogenesis of lung cancer is great; yet the carcinogenic effect appears to be mediated through the action of weak carcinogens. It is imperative to distinguish between minimal concentrations of so-called potent carcinogens and carcinogens of innate weakness.

The significance for man of most carcinogens identified de novo in the laboratory is a major area of ignorance. We know little of their total contribution to the carcinogenic milieu in which we reside and less of their effect on humans. Laboratories devoted to investigating carcinogenesis are increasing, and the number of carcinogenic agents identified by bioassay is increasing remarkably. Compounds are being bioassayed on the basis of epidemiologic suspicion, as in the past; but in addition chemicals are being selected for study on the basis of structural characteristics, chemical relationship to known carcinogenic agents, and low-grade chronic toxicity. There is an urgent need for epidemiological studies to establish the role, if any, of the hundreds of laboratory carcinogens in the panorama of cancer incidence.

The problems of multiple exposure and the relationship of non-carcinogenic environmental agents to the action of carcinogens are numerous; the role of multiple factors cannot be questioned. Laboratory demonstration and quantification of this phenomenon has its clinical counterpart in human cancer; e.g. the high risk to lung cancer noted in asbestos workers, uranium miners and coke oven operators is further enhanced by cigarette smoking. Interference with the metabolism of carcinogenic polycyclic aromatic hydrocarbons, and consequently increased tumor yield, as a result of transient, mild hepatic injury has clinical counterparts. The frequency of both smoking and alcohol consumption in individuals may have a significant implication for the carcinogenic risk associated with exposure to each.

We still do not know whether there exists a threshold of response to chemical carcinogens. Traditional pharmacological dose-response relationships can be elegantly described in the laboratory but only crudely in man. The many sources of environmental carcinogenic agents, their interaction and multiple roles in etiology, and the long latent period required for tumor induction make the determination of threshold and dose response a laboratory undertaking of major importance.

CONCLUSION

The large and heterogeneous array of stimuli that can cause cancer, experimental laboratory data on carcinogenesis, and the varied epidemiologic pattern of cancer unite to support several conclusions:

1. Exposure to carcinogens occurs in a highly complex environment in which multiple factors can be identified as potentially affecting the presence of and response to carcinogenic stimuli.

2. Quantitative studies in model systems demonstrate the interaction of multiple carcinogenic stimuli in inducing cancer.

3. Geographic, occupational, general environmental, cultural, and ethnic

characteristics of population groups having unique cancer risks suggest that their pattern of risk results from simultaneous or sequential action of a combination of environmental and host factors.

CHAPTER 3. POTENTIAL CONTRIBUTIONS OF MULTIPLE RISK FACTORS TO THE ETIOLOGY OF CIRRHOSIS

Thomas C. Chalmers, Clinical Center,
National Institutes of Health, Bethesda, Maryland

It is traditional to think of each case of cirrhosis of the liver as the end result of one of several independent etiologies, known and unknown. If the patient has consumed inordinate amounts of alcohol in his lifetime, he has alcoholic cirrhosis; if he has suffered an attack of acute hepatitis in his youth or at the onset of his present illness, he is diagnosed with confidence as post-hepatitic cirrhosis; if the cirrhosis is preceded by chronic active hepatitis, his disease is considered to be either a chronic viral infection or auto-immune in etiology; if none of these factors is present in his history, his disease is labeled cryptogenic cirrhosis.

A combination of two or more of the above factors, or of one of the above plus as yet undescribed genetic or environmental influences, is rarely considered. The reason is obvious. It is hard enough to establish or rule out any one known factor, much less incriminate more than one. Yet there are some epidemiologic and experimental data to suggest that cirrhosis may, like coronary artery disease, result from the interplay of multiple risk factors. It is the purpose of this paper to examine the validity of the more common single etiologies and speculate about how they may be combined to hasten the disease in certain susceptibles.

ALCOHOLIC CIRRHOSIS

The fact that excessive consumption of alcoholic beverages causes cirrhosis of the liver in some susceptibles has been known for centuries. William Heberden (1710-1801) said "Men are more commonly affected with cirrhous livers than women, because they are more given to intemperate drinking, which is the principal cause of this disorder." (1) The frequency and mechanisms by which alcohol damages the liver in man are still a matter of dispute. The evidence that it does so is of two kinds.

CLINICAL OBSERVATIONS -- It is a common clinical impression that the steady consumer of alcohol, rather than the spree drinker, more frequently develops cirrhosis. The data in Table 1 were gathered by the author 25 years ago before he appreciated the importance of observer bias, but they are suggestive and have not been refuted. The steady drinker eats moderately well, although he usually skips breakfast, until the anorexia of cirrhosis supervenes and in his misery he turns to an all liquid diet. He has rarely had DT's or been jailed for alcoholism, common characteristics of the spree drinker who eats nothing and drinks much more during a spree. The incipient development of cirrhosis in a functioning man or woman who is not obviously an alcoholic is an important concept because intervention may save that person from irreversible cirrhosis. It is also an important concept because other as yet unidentified factors may determine whether or not the individual develops cirrhosis and turns to full-blown alcoholism as his only means of remaining comfortable.

TABLE 1 -- INCIDENCE OF SPREE AND STEADY DRINKING
HABITS IN ALCOHOLIC PATIENTS
(Boston City Hospital Series)

	Cirrhosis	No Known Cirrhosis
Total No.	132	115
Spree %	5.3	43.5
Mixed %	9.1	14.8
Steady %	85.6	41.7

Aside from the regularity of alcohol consumption, the absolute amount is undoubtedly important. Péquignot (2) carried out a careful comparison of the alcohol consumption of a group of cirrhotics and suitable controls (Table 2). The two groups apparently differed only with regard to their alcohol consumption. Their diets were about the same. It should be noted that there was a fair amount of overlap. Lelbach (3) found a reasonable dividing line and emphasized that the consumption was usually excessive for 15 to 20 years before the patient developed cirrhosis. Again there was enough variability for other factors to have been at play.

EPIDEMIOLOGIC DATA -- Jolliffe and Jellinek (4) were the first to summarize effectively the epidemiologic bits of evidence in favor of alcoholism as a principal cause of cirrhosis. Briefly, these are a highly significant association of alcohol consumption per unit of population by state or nation and death rate from cirrhosis, and the changes over time of cirrhosis death rates in a number of countries with the apparent availability of alcohol (4,5,6,7,8). In the United States, France, and Britain, the cirrhosis death rates fell sharply during World War I, and in the United States the rate did not start a steady climb to the present until the repeal of Prohibition. In all three the rates fell again during World War II, rose promptly in the USA and, after a brief lag, rose again to new heights in France, but have stayed down in Britain. Lilienfeld and Korns (6) have objected to these data as clearly indicating alcohol consumption as the sole cause of the reported changes in cirrhosis death rates. They suggest that the absence of a rise in rates for non-whites after the repeal of Prohibition and the

TABLE 2 -- ALCOHOL INTAKE IN GRAMS PER DAY
OF 265 CIRRHOTICS AND CONTROLS (2)

Alcohol Consumption Grams per Day	Per cent of Subjects	
	Cirrhotics	Controls
<80	5	55
80-160	34	36
>160	61	9

preponderance of cirrhosis among urban white males suggest an occupational element. Fifteen years later Terris (7) reported that the rates among non-whites and women have risen and attributes the tardiness to economic factors. He also emphasizes that the urban occupations with the highest rates are those with the easiest access to alcoholic beverages (Table 3). An interesting quirk of economic influence is illustrated by the fact that in Britain, where alcohol is extremely dear as a result of taxation, the professionals and business men have the highest cirrhosis rates, whereas in the United States, where alcohol is cheap, the lowest economic classes have the highest rates (Table 4). So there is no gainsaying the importance of alcohol addiction as a cause of cirrhosis in man. There remains the challenge of explaining the obvious variation in the amount of alcohol necessary to cause cirrhosis. Is this due to historical inaccuracies, or are there identifiable genetic, dietary, or environmental factors that determine which consumer of alcohol develops cirrhosis? These will be considered after the other potential single causes of cirrhosis have been reviewed.

"POST-HEPATITIC" CIRRHOSIS

Four types of data have been employed to associate or obviate acute viral hepatitis as a cause of cirrhosis:

ANECDOTAL DATA -- A number of patients have been described whose livers progressed morphologically from the picture of acute viral hepatitis to

TABLE 3 -- OCCUPATION GROUPS WITH THE HIGHEST STANDARDIZED MORTALITY RATIOS FOR CIRRHOSIS (7)

	S.M.R.
Waiters, Bartenders	392
Longshoremen and stevedores	342
Bakers	219
Laundry and dry cleaning	206
Managers, trades	145
Salesmen and clerks	127

TABLE 4 -- DISTRIBUTION OF CIRRHOSIS STANDARDIZED
MORTALITY RATIOS BY OCCUPATION (7)

		United States	United Kingdom
I.	Professional workers	90	207
II.	Intermediate occupations	88	152
III.	Skilled occupations	105	84
IV.	Semiskilled workers	118	70
V.	Unskilled laborers	148	96

non-alcoholic cirrhosis (9,10). However, none of these have occurred during established epidemics of IH (Virus A) disease, except for a sex-linked episode in post-war Scandinavia (11).

SEROLOGIC DATA -- Hepatitis-associated antigen has been found more frequently in patients with chronic active hepatitis and non-alcoholic cirrhosis than in those with any other disease (Table 5). However, the high rates in Down's syndrome, leukemia, and leprosy suggest that the agent does not necessarily cause all diseases with which it is associated, and, since about 20% of normal adults have antibodies indicating prior infection with HAA, the agent may reappear in the blood as a secondary manifestation of the disease. This is an alternate, if unlikely, explanation for the association.

EPIDEMIOLOGIC DATA -- There are now five cohort studies comparing the incidence of cirrhosis five to twenty years after acute viral hepatitis (largely but not exclusively IH or Virus A disease among military personnel) totaling 7,665 hepatitis patients followed (9,12) with suitable controls. There are less cases of cirrhosis among the hepatitis patients. So that, if epidemic viral hepatitis causes cirrhosis, it does so very, very rarely. Furthermore, there seems to be no increased incidence of cirrhosis among populations of institutionalized retarded children, most of whom become infected with both types of hepatitis virus.

EXPERIMENTAL DATA -- There is as yet no evidence of cirrhosis in the only animals infected with a human hepatitis virus -- marmosets and chimpanzees.

TABLE 5 -- FREQUENCY OF AU ANTIGENEMIA IN VARIOUS
CHRONIC DISEASES

Disease	No. of Reports	No. Examined	No. Au +	% Au +
Cirrhosis				
Non-alcoholic	16	578	66	11.4
Alcoholic	9	323	1	0.3
Unspecified, mixed and other chronic liver diseases	10	806	31	3.8
Hepatitis				
Chronic persistent	12	414	85	20.5
Chronic active	22	760	145	19.7
Down's Syndrome	9	1185	408	34.4
Hemophilias	2	99	5	5.0
Leprosy	1	1189	81	6.8
Leukemia	2	209	19	9.0
Liver neoplasms	7	306	13	4.2

However, a chronic hepatitis has been created in dogs
by partially immunizing them against canine hepatitis
virus (13).

"AUTO-IMMUNE" CIRRHOSIS

Auto-immune factors have been implicated as a
cause of cirrhosis for more than a decade (14). The
concept is based largely on the presence in many
patients, especially females, of hyper-gamma
globulinemia and antibodies to various tissue factors
such as smooth muscle, DNA, and mitochondria
(15,16). However, it has still not been demonstrated
that these abnormal phenomena are primary rather than
secondary. Only in primary biliary cirrhosis has an
antigen-antibody complex been demonstrated in hepatic
cells. It is intriguing, however, that women, who
have chronic "auto-immune" hepatitis and cirrhosis
more often than men, have more antibody to HAA than
men, while the latter have more antigen than women.
The recent observation that a cathartic, previously
demonstrated to cause an acute hepatitis of a
hypersensitivity type, can also cause chronic
hepatitis and cirrhosis (17) is an exciting example
of an immunologic basis of chronic liver disease.

TOXIC CIRRHOSIS

Carbon tetrachloride-induced cirrhosis has long been assumed to occur in chronically exposed humans, and has been produced experimentally in animals (18). More recently, toxins produced by fungi, of which aflatoxin is the best known example, have been shown to produce cirrhosis, albeit rarely, in animals (19), and have been associated epidemiologically in some parts of the world (20). A surprisingly large number of plants and fungi have been associated with the production of cirrhosis in animals, and possibly also in man (21).

OTHER FACTORS THAT MAY FACILITATE THE DEVELOPMENT OF CIRRHOSIS

DIETARY DEFICIENCIES -- Although there are no examples of the production of cirrhosis by dietary factors alone, and dietary deficiency as an important contributor to experimental alcoholic cirrhosis in rats remains a matter of dispute (22,23), the probability remains that the poor diet of many alcoholics contributes to the development of their disease. It is certainly an important factor in any chronic liver disease when anorexia becomes severe.

GENETIC FACTORS -- Lack of body hair (24), color blindness, and aberrant ABO blood group distributions (25) have been cited as evidence that genetic predisposition plays a part in the genesis of cirrhosis. These data are not very impressive, and it is impossible to separate cirrhotic from alcoholic associations. However, the finding of an increased frequency of so-called auto-antibodies in the relatives of patients with non-alcoholic cirrhosis suggests that genetic factors may be involved in susceptibility to this disease (26). Familial cirrhosis with none of the stigmata of Wilson's disease has been described (27).

GEOGRAPHIC FACTORS AND RELATION TO HEPATOMA -- Hepatoma and non-alcoholic cirrhosis occur together and separately with increased frequency in many parts of the world, and this is especially true in the Far East and Africa. The etiologic aspects of geographic factors have been reviewed by Steiner (28) and by Higginson (29), but they don't help very much from the standpoint of multiple etiologies, except to suggest that hepatitis, parasites, and toxins may all play a part in the underdeveloped nations.

AIR POLLUTION -- Recently a study carried out in Buffalo, New York, has suggested that the cirrhosis rates are highest in those sections of the city with the greatest particulate matter in the air and that the differences are not explained by economic factors (30). This is an exciting idea and harks back to the suggestion of Lilienfeld and Korns (6) that incidence might be more frequent in the inner city because of the possibility of toxins in the atmosphere. However, this idea is contradicted by a study of Ayer and Lynch (31). Occupational hazards in their study were rated by public health officers with regard to four kinds of potential toxicity; the degree of exposure to four types of toxins was compared with the severity of three chronic diseases, emphysema, carcinoma of the lung, and cirrhosis. There was a significant negative association between exposure to particulate matter and cirrhosis, probably resulting from the fact that alcoholics did not qualify for jobs of that type. An intriguing environmental factor leading to increased cirrhosis in the inner city is suggested by an experiment of Pogrund (32) showing that rats chronically exposed to 200 parts per million of carbon monoxide, approximately that found on a busy city street, drank significantly more alcohol in place of drinking water than suitable controls (Table 6). The data in this study have not yet been confirmed or explained.

TABLE 6 -- PREFERENCE OF RATS CHRONICALLY EXPOSED TO CARBON MONOXIDE, 200 PPM, FOR ALCOHOL (32)

Day from start of exposure	Volume of fluid in ml. per rat					
	5% Ethanol		3% Glucose		0.3% Cyclamate	
	Air	CO	Air	CO	Air	CO
5	45	32	25	62	23	36
15	62	55	82	66	26	45
30	63	85	66	62	52	45
45	70	140	63	65	34	42
60	40	182	55	62	45	49

A POSSIBLE MECHANISM TO EXPLAIN COMBINED EFFECTS

In general, there is a tremendous mushrooming of papers on the stimulation of various enzyme systems in the liver and its effect on the degradation and toxicity of foreign substances. For instance, it has now become apparent that carbon tetrachloride toxicity can be markedly increased, and the development of cirrhosis accelerated, by stimulation of the endoplasmic reticulum by phenobarbitone. Presumably, the stimulated enzymes are then converting the toxin to a more toxic substance (33,34). DDT has been shown to stimulate hepatic enzymes and increased carbon tetrachloride toxicity. A number of other substances are toxic to the liver only after they have been converted by enzymes to toxic elements (35). It is thus entirely possible, but highly speculative, that chronic exposure to various noxious elements which stimulate the endoplasmic reticulum of the liver at the same time increase the susceptibility of the liver to other toxins -- a truly potential combination of etiologic agents in the pathogenesis of cirrhosis. Unfortunately, the only work on alcoholic damage in animals suggests that stimulation of the enzymes diminish that damage, rather than increase it (36). An explanation for tolerance to alcohol among people taking phenobarbital may lie in stimulation of the enzyme necessary to metabolize acetaldehyde (37). These data need to be confirmed and expanded.

COMBINATIONS OF TWO OR MORE OF THE ABOVE FACTORS

It is most intriguing to speculate that cirrhosis may occur as the end result of a combination of two or more of the above factors, just as multiple risk factors have been established as contributing in a cumulative way to the risk of coronary artery disease. However, no such data are available for cirrhosis. The rates of prior hepatitis and of HA antigenemia are about the same in patients with alcoholic cirrhosis as in the normal population. Although some alcoholic cirrhotics have high gamma globulins and occasional positive antibody tests, there is no evidence that a familial or sex-related tendency to respond in this manner has made them likely to develop cirrhosis on a smaller than average alcohol intake. Data on alcohol intake are too unreliable to rule the possibility in or out.

It is conceivable, however, that some of the peanuts served in bars could be contaminated with aflatoxin. Even though it is so hard to prove, either in humans or experimental animals, it is entirely possible that the variability in susceptibility to cirrhosis among alcoholics, or to various other toxins among non-alcoholics, is the result of a combination of risk factors such as genetic predisposition and stimulation of hepatic enzymes by various unsuspected environmental substances. This should be a fruitful area for future research.

REFERENCES

1. Heberden, W. (1710-1801). Commentary on the History and Cure of Diseases (London 1802). Quoted in Strauss, M. B. (1968). Familiar Medical Quotations. Little, Brown, Boston, p. 276.

2. Péquignot, G. (1963). Do questionnaire surveys enable us to determine the incidence of the alcoholic etiology of liver cirrhosis? Bull. Acad. Natl. Méd. 147: 90.

3. Leibach, W. K. (1966). Leberschäden bei chronischem Alkoholismus. Ergebnisse einer klinischen, klinischchemischen und bioptisch-histologischen Untersuchung an 526 Alkoholkranken während der Entziehungskur in einer offenen Trinkerheilstätte. Acta Hepato-splenol (Stuttg.) 13: 321.

4. Jolliffe, N. and Jellinek, E. M. (1941). Vitamin deficiencies and liver cirrhosis in alcoholism. Part VII. Cirrhosis of the liver. Q. J. Stud. Alcohol 2: 544.

5. Martini, G. A. and Bode, C. (1970). Epidemiology of liver cirrhosis. Internist 11: 84.

6. Lilienfeld, A. M. and Korns, R. F. (1950). Some epidemiological aspects of cirrhosis of the liver. A study of mortality statistics. Amer. J. Hyg. 52: 65.

7. Terris, M. (1967). Epidemiology of cirrhosis of the liver: National mortality data. Amer. J. Public Health 57: 2076.

8. Creutzfeldt, W. and Beck, K. (1966). Cirrhosis of the liver: on the aetiology, pathogenesis, results of treatment and period of survival in an unselected series of 560 patients. Dtsch. Med. Wschr. 91: 682.

9. Chalmers, T. C. and Sebestyen, C. S. (1963). Evidence against infectious hepatitis as a cause of cirrhosis. Trans. Amer. Clin. Climatol. Assoc. 74: 192.

10. Klatskin, G. (1958). Subacute hepatic necrosis and postnecrotic cirrhosis due to anicteric infections with the hepatitis virus. Amer. J. Med. 25: 333.

11. Jersild, M. (1947). Infectious hepatitis with subacute atrophy of the liver. An epidemic in women after menopause. New Eng. J. Med. 237: 6.

12. Beebe, G. W. and Simon, A. H. (1970). Cirrhosis of the liver following viral hepatitis, a twenty-year mortality follow-up. Amer. J. Epidemiol. 92: 279.

13. Gocke, D. J., Morris, T. Q. and Bradley, S. E. (1970). Chronic hepatitis in the dog: The role of immune factors. J. Amer. Vet. Med. Assoc. 156: 1700.

14. Goldgraber, M. B. and Kirsner, J. B. (1961). The hypersensitive state and the liver: A critical review. Amer. J. Med. Sci. 241: 109.

15. Doniach, D. and Walker, J. G. (1969). A unified concept of autoimmune hepatitis. Lancet 1: 813.

16. Doniach, D. et al. (1970). "Autoallergic" hepatitis. New Eng. J. Med. 282: 86.

17. Reynolds, T. B., Yamada, S. and Peters, R. L. (1971). Chronic active and lupoid hepatitis due to a laxative, oxyphenisatin. Gastroenterology 60: 750.

18. Cameron, G. R. and Karunaratne, W. A. E. (1936). Carbon tetrachloride cirrhosis in relation to liver regeneration. J. Pathol. Bacteriol. 42: 1.

19. Butler, W. H. (1970). Liver injury induced by aflatoxin. In: H. Popper and F. Schaffner, (eds.). Progress in Liver Diseases, III. Grune and Stratton, New York and London, 408.

20. Amla, I. et al. (Unpublished data). Lesions identical to Indian childhood cirrhosis resulting from consumption of aflatoxin contaminated peanut protein supplement in children suffering from protein malnutrition.

21. Davidson, C. S. (1963). Plants and fungi as etiologic agents of cirrhosis. New Eng. J. Med. 268: 1072.

22. Rubin, E. and Lieber, C. S. (1968). Malnutrition and liver disease -- an overemphasized relationship (Editorial). Amer. J. Med. 45: 1.

23. Porta, E. A. et al. (1967). Dietary factors in the progression and regression of hepatic alterations associated with experimental chronic alcoholism. Fed. Proc. 26: 1449.

24. Lloyd, C. W. and Williams, R. H. (1948). Endocrine changes associated with Laennec's cirrhosis of the liver. Amer. J. Med. 4: 315.

25. Reid, N. C. R. W. et al. (1968). Genetic characteristics and cirrhosis: A controlled study of 200 patients. Brit. Med. J. 2: 463.

26. Elling, P., Ranløv, P. and Bildsøe, P. (1966). A genetic approach to the pathogenesis of

hepatic cirrhosis. A clinical and serological study. Acta Med. Scand. 179: 527.

27. Iber, F. L. and Maddrey, W. C. (1966). Familial hepatic diseases with portal hypertension with or without cirrhosis. In: H. Popper and F. Schaffner, (eds.). Progress in Liver Diseases, II. Grune and Stratton, New York and London, 290.

28. Steiner, P. E. (1964). World problem in the cirrhotic diseases of the liver: Their incidence, frequency, types and aetiology. Trop. Geogr. Med. 16: 175.

29. Higginson, J. (1966). Geographic considerations in liver disease. In: H. Popper and F. Schaffner, (eds.). Progress in Liver Diseases, II. Grune and Stratton, New York and London, 211.

30. Winkelstein, W. and Gay, M. L. (1971). Suspended particulate air pollution: Relationship to mortality from cirrhosis of the liver. Arch. Env. Health 22: 175.

31. Ayer, H. E. and Lynch, J. R. (1968). Association of disability and selected occupational hazards. Arch. Env. Health 17: 225.

32. Pogrund, R. S. (1969). Biologic synergisms in rats produced by carbon monoxide and positive ions. Int. J. Biometeorol. 13: 123.

33. McLean, E. K., McLean, A. E. M. and Sutton, P. M. (1969). Instant cirrhosis. An improved method for producing cirrhosis of the liver in rats by simultaneous administration of carbon tetrachloride and phenobarbitone. Brit. J. Exp. Pathol. 50: 502.

34. McLean, A. E. M. (1970). The effect of protein deficiency and microsomal enzyme induction by DDT and phenobarbitone on the acute toxicity of chloroform and a pyrrolizidine alkaloid, retrorsine. Brit. J. Exp. Pathol. 51: 317.

35. McLean, A. E. M. (1970). Conversion by the liver of inactive molecules into toxic molecules. In: W. N. Aldridge, (ed.) Mechanisms of Toxicity, Biological Council Symposium. MacMillan and Company, London, 219.

36. Koff, R. S. et al. (1970). Prevention of the ethanol-induced fatty liver in the rat by phenobarbital. Gastroenterology 59: 50.

37. Redmond, G. and Cohen, G. (1971). Induction of liver acetaldehyde dehydrogenase: Possible role in ethanol tolerance after exposure to barbiturates. Science 171: 387.

CHAPTER 4. MULTIPLE FACTOR ETIOLOGY IN CORONARY HEART DISEASE

Jerome Cornfield, Federation of American Societies
of Experimental Biology, Bethesda, Maryland

Virtually all of our current quantitative knowledge on the multiple etiology of coronary heart disease has been provided by epidemiological investigation during the last twenty years. I shall first sketch the general nature of this knowledge and then go on to indicate the nature of efforts now in progress to see whether applications of this knowledge to prevention and control are possible.

INTERNATIONAL COMPARISONS

The most elementary, and perhaps impressive, evidence that modifiable environmental factors may be important determinants of mortality from coronary heart disease is provided by international comparisons of native-born and migrant populations (1). Table 1 shows age-specific mortality from coronary heart disease among U.S. white men in 1960 to 1961 and compares it with data from Denmark, Norway, and Sweden. Below age 55, the Scandinavian rates are less than one-half of ours; between 55 to 74, about 40% less; and even above age 75, about 20% less. That these differences are not artifacts due to international differences in certification of causes of death is indicated by comparison of mortality from all causes (Table 2). Although somewhat reduced, the percentage differences are still apparent at all ages below 75.

In contrast, we have the mortality experience of native-born Scandinavians who migrated to the United States and were presumably exposed to a new range and intensity of environmental variables. Their

TABLE 1 -- ANNUAL NO. OF DEATHS/100,000 POPULATION
FROM ARTERIOSCLEROTIC AND DEGENERATIVE
HEATH DISEASE (B26) IN SELECTED COUNTRIES,
BY AGE, WHITE MALES, 1960-61

Age Groups (yrs.)	United States	Denmark	Norway	Sweden
0-24	0.5	0.6	0.2	0.1
25-34	10.8	5.3	5.5	2.7
35-44	89.2	29.8	30.5	20.5
45-54	361.4	149.3	157.3	115.1
55-64	931.9	496.3	499.6	485.5
65-74	2034.6	1294.3	1173.3	1344.7
75+	4893.6	3773.6	2997.6	4113.3

TABLE 2 -- ANNUAL NO. OF DEATHS/100,000 POPULATION
FROM ALL CAUSES IN SELECTED COUNTRIES,
BY AGE, WHITE MALES, 1960-61

Age Groups (yrs.)	United States	Denmark	Norway	Sweden
0-24	219.5	171.0	173.7	139.6
25-34	160.9	121.6	135.5	125.0
35-44	329.3	207.8	228.9	207.2
45-54	916.4	580.4	527.6	508.0
55-64	2194.3	1574.5	1482.5	1443.8
65-74	4795.4	3931.4	3591.4	3864.7
75+	11837.9	11919.6	11457.8	11820.4

mortality experience was much closer to, and for some age groups indistinguishable from, that of native-born Americans (Table 3). We cannot definitely exclude the possibility that these differences simply reflect selective factors which determine who migrates and who stays home. But migrants, if anything, are selected for lower and not higher mortality. The most plausible explanation of these differences is exposure to a less favorable set of environmental determinants with respect to coronary disease in the United States in contrast to the country of origin. The results of the

44

TABLE 3 -- ANNUAL NO. OF DEATHS/100,000 POPULATION
FROM CORONARY HEART DISEASE (ISC 420 &
422) AND FROM ALL CAUSES AMONG MALE
NORWEGIAN AND SWEDISH* IMMIGRANTS LIVING
IN THE UNITED STATES, BY AGE, 1959-61

Age Groups	Coronary Heart Disease Deaths		Deaths from All Causes	
	Born in Norway	Born in Sweden	Born in Norway	Born in Sweden
25-34	9.7	--	194.1	178.4
35-44	78.2	39.1	368.9	234.4
45-54	281.0	327.3	892.3	890.0
55-64	762.4	817.3	1961.0	2016.4
64-74	1890.4	2003.0	4483.2	4810.7
75+	5937.2	5659.3	14334.2	13943.0

* Mortality for Danish-born living in the United
States has not been tabulated.

Source: U.S. National Center for Health Statistics

British-Norwegian migrant study, which, when
available, will compare the mortality of migrants to
the United States with that of siblings who did not
migrate, should cast further light on this question.
If the differences between Scandinavians living in
Scandinavia and those migrating to the United
States are environmentally mediated, then to the
extent that the United States and Scandinavia
present environmental risks in common, the
magnitude of environmental effects are
underestimated by this comparison.

RISK FACTORS IN FRAMINGHAM

When we turn to the findings of longitudinal
studies, we see results consistent with this
interpretation, as well as suggestions as to
which specific environmental factors might be
involved. These findings may be quantitated by using
the recent multivariate analysis of risk factors in
Framingham (2), and by restricting attention to
the four potentially modifiable risk factors shown
in Table 4:

TABLE 4 -- TWELVE-YEAR RISK OF CORONARY HEART DISEASE
FOR DIFFERING LEVELS RISK FACTORS BY AGE,
FRAMINGHAM MALES, 1948-60 (2)

Serum Cholesterol (X_1)		Systolic Blood Pressure (X_2)		Rel. Wt. (X_3)		Smoking (X_4)		New Events/ 1,000 by Entrance Age (yrs.) 35	45	55
250		150		110		1 pack		67	209	261
	220	150		110		1 pack		35	175	212
	220		130	110		1 pack		23	152	164
	220		130		100	1 pack		20	120	154
	220		130		100		0 pack	6	54	95

Age group
at Exam 1

30-39 $y=\log_e[P/(1-P)]=-17.6+.023X_1+.022X_2+.014X_3+.598X_4+.092X_5$
40-49 $y=\log_e[P/(1-P)]=-13.7+.007X_1+.009X_2+.027X_3+.434X_4+.120X_5$
50-62 $y=\log_e[P/(1-P)]=-11.1+.009X_1+.016X_2+.008X_3+.272X_4+.072X_5$

(X_1) Serum cholesterol (mg/100 ml)

(X_2) Systolic blood pressure (mmHg)

(X_3) Relative weight (100 X actual weight ÷ median weight for sex-height group)

(X_4) Cigarette smoking, coded as

   0 = Never smoked
   1 = Less than a pack a day
   2 = One pack a day
   3 = More than one pack a day.

The Framingham experience is summarized in the equations for the three age groups listed, at the bottom of Table 4. P is the 12-year probability of new coronary heart disease; X_1 through X_4 stand for possible values of the risk factors in the order already listed and at the top of Table 4; and X_5 is age in years. These equations provide a compact and faithful summary description of the relations found in Framingham. To find the 12-year probability associated with given values of the four risk factors for a designated age, substitute the four values into the appropriate equation to obtain the logit of risk, y. The probability itself is then computed as $1/(1 + e^{-y})$, where e is 2.71828.

Table 4 gives some idea of the information that can be extracted from these equations. For each of the three age groups we have started with a hypothetical individual with a serum cholesterol value of 250, blood pressure of 150, a relative weight of 110, and smoking one pack of cigarettes a day. Calculated risks expressed as number of new events in 12 yr/1,000 exposed are then 67 at age 35, 209 at age 45, and 261 at age 55. These correspond to about the ninth decile of risk at each of the three age groups. If now we hold the last three risk factors at their initial values, but recalculate using serum cholesterol values of 220 rather than 250, we obtain the lowered Framingham risk associated with this lower cholesterol value. At age 35 the estimated risk is lowered from 67 to 35, or about 50%, as compared with a reduction of about 20% at the higher age groups. If, in addition, we use blood pressures of 130 rather than 150, the third line of Table 4 results with an additional lowering of one-third.

The magnitudes of the reductions are substantial and well in excess of the United States-Scandinavian differences shown in Tables 1 and 2. The risks associated with the lower values of all four variables are 90% below the starting values at age 35, 75% at age 45, and 65% at age 55. This reduced ability to affect risk at the higher age groups is consistent with the diminishing percentage differences in mortality between the United States and Scandinavia with increasing age. To the extent that either set of data bears on the question of what can be achieved by actually intervening on known risk factors, they support the view that important effects of intervention cannot be expected at higher ages, say above 65, even though this is where the majority of deaths actually occur, but that the possibility exists of achieving substantial effects at earlier ages.

OTHER RISK FACTORS

Although the risk factors analyzed above are among the most important of those that have been

47

epidemiologically implicated, many others, over 35 by one estimate (3), could be listed. The most important single risk factor not included in the above analysis is physical activity, which has been implicated in numerous studies. Results of a recent study by Frank et al. (4) are summarized in Table 5. The physical activity classes of the table are constructed from responses to a questionnaire concerning job-related and nonoccupational activities.

The far from trivial aggregate effect of these other risk factors can be quantified by noting that Framingham men aged 50-62 who were in the lowest decile of risk with respect to these particular risk factors (and in addition the endogenous factor of ECG abnormality), nevertheless had the same expectation of a new coronary event as younger men aged 30-39 in the eighth decile of risk for the younger age group with respect to these same risk factors (2).

Two other recent findings indicate the non-specific nature of the agents that can be involved in the etiology of cardiovascular disease: (a) a positive relation between water softness and cardiovascular mortality (5), and (b) the excess cardiovascular mortality associated with the oral hypoglycemic agents, tolbutamide and phenformin (6,7). The water softness relation was originally reported in Japan and subsequently confirmed in the

TABLE 5 -- INCIDENCE AND EARLY MORTALITY AMONG MEN, 25-64, BY PHYSICAL ACTIVITY AND SMOKING -- AGE ADJUSTED (4)

Physical activity	No. of men	1st Myocardial Infarctions Rate per 1000 per year	% dying in 4 weeks	4 week death rate per 1000 per year
Cigarette smokers				
Least active	47	7.4	50	3.7
Intermediate	68	5.1	33	1.7
Most active	67	5.7	22	1.2
Non-Cigarette smokers				
Least active	39	5.2	56	2.9
Intermediate	50	2.9	18	0.5
Most active	28	2.2	15	0.3

48

United States, England and Wales, and to some extent in Sweden. Boroughs in England and Wales with less than 10 ppm of water calcium have a reported elevation in mortality from cardiovascular disease of about 50% compared to those with more than 100 ppm. The biological basis for this relation is not well understood. Since a positive relation, but of reduced magnitude, has also been found for other causes of death, the specificity of the relation for cardiovascular disease is not clearly established. It could simply reflect the peculiarities of the correlation coefficient as a measure of the magnitude of the relation between water softness and the individual causes of death. The cardiogenic effects of the hypoglycemic agents were discovered in a collaborative, long-term, randomized, clinical trial designed to test the possible efficacy of various agents in preventing cardiovascular complications among adult-onset diabetics. Contrary to expectation, the observed effect was to increase mortality and for each agent the decision to discontinue patients assigned to it seemed indicated and was taken. The findings on tolbutamide have not been universally accepted (8).

PRE- AND POST-INFARCT POPULATIONS

The effect of the various risk factors need not be the same in all sub-classes of the population. In particular, early results of the Coronary Drug Project suggest that cigarette smoking and cholesterol levels may be less important as risk factors in men who have survived their first myocardial infarct, than in those not yet experiencing one (9). In Table 6 the pre- and post-infarct experience in Framingham and in the Coronary Drug Project are compared. Although the comparison is clearly in need of considerable refinement, the suggestion of a much reduced relation in the post-infarct population, if indeed there is any at all, is unmistakable. A similar failure of serum cholesterol to predict post-infarct risk of coronary heart disease for men, but not women, has been reported for the Health Insurance Plan (HIP) population (10). More recent, and as yet unpublished, analyses from the Coronary Drug Project show a somewhat sharper relation between serum cholesterol and percent deaths

TABLE 6 -- COMPARISON OF CHOLESTEROL LEVEL AND AMOUNT
SMOKED AS RISK FACTORS IN PRE- AND POST-INFARCT
MALE POPULATIONS (2,9)

A. Cholesterol

Post-infarct (9)		Pre-infarct (2)	
Cholesterol mg/ml	Percent deceased	Cholesterol mg/100 ml	12 yr. incidence coronary events, men, 50-62
< 200	5.0	< 190	10.5
200-249	5.0	{190-219 {220-249	{18.7 {20.0
250-299	6.7		
≥300	6.1	≥250	25.7

B. Smoking

Cigarettes/ day	Percent deceased	Packs/day	12 yr. incidence coronary events, men, 50-62
None	5.1	None	16.9
1-20	6.0	{<1 { 1	{23.8 {18.1
≥21	5.0	>1	27.0

than originally reported, but still below that in
pre-infarct populations.

JOINT EFFECTS

Little published information is available on the
nature of the interaction between the various risk
factors. One might consider in theory the
possibility that one or more particular combinations
are pathognomonic, but information currently
available makes this appear most unlikely. For any
single risk factor there appears to be no threshold
or critical value at which the risk-factor intensity
relation changes abruptly (11), and a similar absence
of a multivariately defined critical value seems
likely.

To further consider the question of joint effects it is necessary to define the scale on which risk is measured (Table 4 and comments). If P denotes the probability of an event in unit time for some well-defined population, then the logit of P, namely $\log_e P/(1-P)$, provides a scale in which the effects of the different risk factors can be treated as additive (2,6,12). That is to say, if the elevation in the logit of P associated with an elevation of one unit in risk factor 1 is β_1 and the elevation for one unit of risk factor 2 is β_2, then the elevation associated with a joint increase of one unit in each of the two risk factors can be treated as $\beta_1+\beta_2$. Or equivalently, the effect on this scale of an elevation in any one risk factor, assuming this type of additivity, is independent of the level of the other risk factors. This assumption is in need of a more critical examination than it has yet received. If age is treated as an omnibus risk factor, it is known (2) that additivity does not apply and that the effect on this scale of each of the risk factors studied decreases with increasing age. An early and incomplete test for the joint effects of cholesterol and blood pressure in Framingham found no departures from additivity (13) even though experiments with dogs did indicate that the rate at which albumin entered the aortic wall was higher for hypertensive than for normotensive dogs (14,15).

INTERVENTION STUDIES

The implications for prevention and control of these epidemiologically established relations must of course be established by other means, namely direct experimental intervention. The most clear-cut results to date have been obtained by intervening on hypertension, as reviewed by Freis (16). Antihypertensive therapy in patients with malignant hypertension was demonstrated over 10 years ago to reduce mortality. More recently such therapy in patients with mild hypertension (diastolic pressures between 115 and 129 mmHg.) has been shown to reduce dramatically the incidence of morbid events, the majority of which were manifestations specifically associated with hypertension. A substantial if somewhat less dramatic effect of this therapy on hypertensive complications was subsequently shown in patients with diastolic blood pressures between 90 and 114 mmHg. (17). Neither series demonstrated any effect on atherosclerotic complications.

Cholesterol lowering can be achieved by diet, by drugs, or by surgery. A number of randomized trials to test the effects of intervention with the first two have been undertaken and reviewed by Cornfield and Mitchell (18). The drug trials are still in progress with no results presently available. The most striking of the many diet interventions has been reported by Leren (19), but because of the small size of the trial and lack of double-blindedness it has been regarded as in need of confirmation (20).

A preliminary effort to investigate the effects of an exercise regimen has been terminated because of grossly inadequate adherence. A randomized trial to investigate the effects of discontinuing cigarette smoking is now in progress among civil servants in London (21), but no results are available to date.

The most recent development in the field of intervention trials is the idea of a multifactor preventive trial, i.e. simultaneous intervention on several risk factors with the hope of demonstrating an overall effect, with a somewhat reduced possibility of partitioning whatever effect is found among the various single factors responsible (22). There are two major reasons for considering such a trial. First, one might expect with a multiple intervention an increased magnitude of effect and consequently reduced requirements for numbers of patients. Secondly, single factor interventions have in many cases led to concomitant changes in other variables; for example, diet changes in the National Diet-Heart Study were accompanied by changes in weight, blood pressure, and amount smoked (23), so that whatever effects are found need not be specific to the single factor on which intervention occurred. Two such studies, one in London and the other in Gothenburg have been initiated.

SUMMARY

It is clear that a wide variety of endogenous and exogenous factors are involved in the etiology of coronary heart disease and that intervention on a wide spectrum of characteristics may be required for optimum prevention and control. With the exception of intervention for hypertension, however, the effectiveness of such intervention still remains to be demonstrated.

REFERENCES

1. Krueger, D. E. and Moriyama, I. M. (1967). Mortality of the foreign born. Amer. J. Public Health 57: 496.

2. Truett, J. Cornfield, J. and Kannel, W. (1967). A multivariate analysis of the risk of coronary heart disease in Framingham. J. Chron. Dis. 20: 511.

3. Simborg, D. W. (1970). The status of risk factors and coronary heart disease. J. Chron. Dis. 22: 515.

4. Frank, C. W. et al. (1966). Myocardial infarction in men. Role of physical activity and smoking in incidence and mortality. J. Amer. Med. Assoc. 198: 1241.

5. Crawford, M. D., Gardner, M. J. and Morris, J. N. (1971). Cardiovascular disease and minerals in drinking water. Brit. Med. Bull. 27: 21.

6. The University Group Diabetes Program. (1970). A study of the effects of hypoglycemic agents on vascular complications in patients with adult-onset diabetes, I. Design, methods, and baseline characteristics, II. Mortality results. Diabetes 19: 747 (suppl. 2).

7. The University Group Diabetes Program. (1970). A study of the effects of hypoglycemic agents on vascular complications in patients with adult-onset diabetes, IV. A preliminary report on phenformin results. J. Amer. Med. Assoc. 214: 1303.

8. Feinstein, A. R. (1971). Clinical biostatistics. VIII. An analytic appraisal of

the University Group Diabetes Program (UGDP) study. Clin. Pharmacol. 12: 167.

9. The Cornary Drug Project Research Group. (1970). Control of hyperlipidemia. 4. Progress in drug trials of secondary prevention with particular reference to the coronary drug project in atherosclerosis. In: R. J. Jones, (ed.). Proc. of the Second International Symposium. Springer-Verlag, New York, Heidelberg, Berlin, 586.

10. Frank, C. W., Weinblatt, E. and Shapiro, S. (1970). Prognostic implications of serum cholesterol in coronary heart disease in atherosclerosis. In: R. J. Jones, (ed.). Proc. of the Second International Symposium. Springer-Verlag, New York, Heidelberg, Berlin, 390.

11. Cornfield, J. (1962). Joint dependence of risk of coronary heart disease on serum cholesterol and systolic blood pressure: A discriminant function analysis. Fed. Proc. 21(4): 58.

12. Walker, S. H. and Duncan, D. B. (1967). Estimation of the probability of an event as a function of several independent variables. Biometrika 54: 167.

13. Cornfield, J., Gordon, T. and Smith, W. W. (1961). Quantal response curves for experimentally uncontrolled variables. Bull. Inter. Stat. Inst. (Tokyo) 38: 97).

14. Duncan, L. E., Cornfield, J. and Buck, K. (1962). The effect of blood pressure on the passage of labelled plasma albumin into canine aortic wall. J. Clin. Invest. 41: 1537.

15. Duncan, L. E., Buck, K. and Lynch, A. (1965). The effect of pressure and stretching on the passage of labelled albumin into canine aortic wall. J. Ather. Res. 5: 69.

16. Freis, E. D. (1970). Control of mild hypertension in atherosclerosis. In: R. J. Jones, (ed.). Proc. of the Second

International Symposium. Springer-Verlag, New York, Heidelberg, Berlin, 595.

17. Veterans Administration Cooperative Study Group with Antihypertensive Agents. (1970). Effects of treatment on morbidity in hypertension. II. Results in patients with diastolic blood pressure averaging 90 through 114 mmHg. J. Amer. Med. Assoc. 213: 1143.

18. Cornfield, J. and Mitchell, S. (1969). Selected risk factors in coronary disease possible intervention effects. Arch. Env. Health 19: 382.

19. Leren, P. (1966). The effect of plasma cholesterol lowering diet in male survivors of myocardial infarction. Norwegian Monogr. Med. Sci., Oslo.

20. Diet-Heart Review Panel of the National Heart Institute. (1969). Mass Field-Trials of the diet-heart question their significance, timeliness, feasibility, and applicability. An assessment of seven proposed experimental designs. Amer. Heart Assoc. Monogr. 28, New York.

21. Reid, Donald. Personal communication.

22. Blackburn, H. (In press). Multifactor Preventive Trials (MPT) in coronary heart disease. Trends in epidemiology. In: Gordon T. Stewart, (ed.). American Lectures in Epidemiology, Community Health and Tropical Medicine. Charles C. Thomas, Springfield, Illinois.

23. National Diet-Heart Study Research Group. (1968). The National Diet-Heart Study first report. American Heart Assoc. Monogr. 18, Circulation 37: 1.

CHAPTER 5. MULTIPLE FACTOR ETIOLOGY IN CHRONIC OBSTRUCTIVE LUNG DISEASE

JEROME KLEINERMAN, Department of Pathology,
St. Luke's Hospital, and Case Western Reserve
University School of Medicine, Cleveland, Ohio

Since the group of chronic obstructive lung diseases includes a large number of conditions, the subject will be kept in bounds by excluding allergic bronchial asthma, asthmatic bronchitis, cystic fibrosis and other forms of bronchiolitis from this discussion, although their presence cannot be excluded with certainty from epidemiologic studies.

The major focus of this discussion will be on the disease states emphysema and chronic bronchitis. It is, however, necessary to clarify certain features of these diseases. Although these disease entities can and do have specific and distinguishing pathologic features, it is more common for them to occur together to some degree. While the nature and site of the obstruction may be considered different in these different disease states, there is still considerable debate concerning the exact anatomic site of the obstruction. While the physiological and clinical definitions of chronic obstructive lung disease turn on the observation of an increased resistance to airflow at the mouth, the anatomic features associated with the disease are more complex.

CHARACTERISTICS

Emphysema has been defined as "an abnormal anatomic enlargement of airspaces, distal to the terminal bronchiole and accompanied by destructive changes." This entity is most commonly observed in two forms, the centriacinar and the panacinar. These

57

differ in the location and extent within the anatomic unit of the lung, the acinus. There is considerable controversy at this time as to whether an associated significant bronchiolitis exists concurrently with emphysema. It is generally agreed that the bronchiole specifically related to each centrilobular lesion is not structurally occluded; however, bronchioles in adjacent loci of non-emphysematous lung, as well as in the emphysematous lesion, may demonstrate bronchiolitis with some luminal compromise. The mucosa in these areas may frequently show goblet cell metaplasia. In regions of severe emphysema, bronchioles may be obliterated or completely destroyed.

The classic lesion in chronic bronchitis, on the other hand, is believed to reside in the larger lobar and sublobar bronchi where luminal compromise is produced by mucous gland hyperplasia and hypertrophy, excessive luminal secretion, congestion and hyperemia and perhaps smooth muscle spasm or hyperplasia. Recent studies have demonstrated that in this disease state the smaller bronchi and bronchioles may likewise be the seat of inflammation and luminal compromise from plugs of mucus or increased smooth muscle tonicity, or mural fibrosis and inflammation.

Thus, the anatomic basis of the obstructive diseases may vary from parenchymal destruction to bronchial and bronchiolar inflammation and fibrosis with hypersecretion, and their separation may not be possible with the use of the simple physiologic tests utilized in epidemiologic studies. However, more sophisticated pulmonary function tests may help to differentiate these disease states. These tests include the diffusing capacity of the lung for CO, which signals the loss of available diffusing surface of capillary bed, decreasing dynamic compliance with increasing frequency of respiration, which evaluates the conductivity of small airways at varying respiratory frequencies. Flow-volume loops during passive and forced expiratory efforts permit estimation of the "up-stream" resistance of the distal small airways. Nevertheless, the striking differences in the anatomic features of obstructive disease certainly suggest, not only that they constitute different disease states, but that multiple etiologic factors are at work in the production of such diverse pathology.*

PREVALENCE

If we then satisfy ourselves with the physiologic definition of obstructive disease states utilizing objective tests, what do we know of the prevalence of these disease states in our population? Such a study was performed in 1963 by Prindle and associates (1). In this study the populations of two adjacent towns were surveyed for the prevalence of obstructive lung disease. The primary purpose was to observe the difference in prevalence of chronic obstructive lung disease between a town subjected to chronic air pollution from the effluent of a fossil fuel burning power plant and a town without such pollution. A very slightly higher prevalence of chronic obstructive lung disease was observed in the polluted town as compared to the unpolluted one. Perhaps more important for the purposes of this discussion are the data relating to the prevalence in one of these towns. The objective data (1a), particularly pulmonary function tests, were evaluated to establish norms and standard deviations. They included maximal breathing capacity (MBC), residual volume (RV), and mixing index (MI). 59.8% of a population of 360 males, 30 years old and over, fell within ± 2 S.D. of the mean. 7.6% had all three pulmonary function tests outside of 2 S.D. of the mean; and when every combination of two abnormal (more than 2 S.D. removed from the mean) pulmonary function tests were combined, the total reached over 18%. If additional questionable cases are added to this total, about 20% of the population can be said to have had objective evidence of obstructive disease. These figures are probably a realistic approximation of the incidence of chronic obstructive lung disease in a small urban area, at least in the male population over 30 years of age. They do not, however, give an indication of the prevalence in the female population, nor do they indicate the

---

* For more detailed discussion see "Environmental Factors in Respiratory Disease" in this Series. (Eds.)

prevalence of subclinical or preclinical disease states.**

To gain some insight into this problem, we must use yet another method. The observation of subclinical disease must depend on amplification of the underlying disease state by provocative testing in an available suspect population. A second means, is to look for evidence of specific pathologic changes in a predisease population. This we have done over the past three years by examining: (a) a young population primarily from ages 15-45; and, more recently, (b) older individuals that had died acutely, and usually by violence or suicide; for the presence of emphysema and bronchitis lesions in the lung. In our preliminary study, we evaluated over 115 lungs by hemidecade from 15 to 45 years of age. When the smallest emphysema lesion observed pathologically was taken as evidence of some disease, we noted over 25% of persons in the 15-20 year group with some lesions. The incidence rose to over 80% by age 30. The prevalence of lesions was closely associated with the presence and extent of pigment deposition in the pleura and parenchyma.

In a subsequent study, in addition to observation of lung tissue for emphysema and bronchitis lesions, we attempted to interview the next-of-kin of the deceased for historical information relating to smoking history, family history, site of residence, occupation, previous medical history and other factors which might throw light on correlated factors in the etiology of these lesions. This study is still in progress and to date we have attempted only a preliminary analysis of the data. There is indication that emphysema lesions do exist at an early age. When the extent of the anatomic emphysema observed is separated into categories (0, 1-10%, over 10%) there is good correlation with smoking history, extent of air pollution exposure and age. There is limited

---

** It should be noted that Prindle et al. were unable to include data on smoking and occupational (mostly mining) history and characterized their report as "preliminary". (Eds.)

correlation with occupational exposure and none with social class. Chronic bronchitis similarly evaluated correlates well with smoking history and social class, moderately with air pollution index and occupational exposure. These observations may aid in the understanding of the natural biology of the obstructive disease lesions, and indicate that even in early lesions, probably in the preclinical stage, a multiplicity of factors may be involved in the inception and progression of these diseases.

SMOKING AS ETIOLOGIC AGENT

The evidence that cigarette smoking is an important factor in the causation of chronic obstructive lung disease is adequately documented in the report of the Advisory Committee to the Surgeon General of the Public Health Service, entitled, "Smoking and Health" (2). It is reasonably clear, however, that the occurrence of bronchitis in smokers is not a universal finding and, while the prevalence of this disease and emphysema is greater in the smoking population, it is also present to a lesser extent in the non-smoking population. This suggests that smoking is but one of the factors in the genesis of obstructive pulmonary diseases. It is important also to distinguish between the acute and chronic effects of smoking. It has been documented by Nadel and Comroe (3) that, following the inhalation of cigarette smoke, both smokers and non-smokers respond acutely by a marked decrease of airway conductance of 31%. A similar change in these parameters can be observed from the inhalation of chemically inert fine particles. This has been substantiated by other workers (4). Studies of chronic smokers have likewise demonstrated changes in the pulmonary function particularly in the presence of functional abnormalities of residual volume, lung mixing, diffusing capacity and airway resistance. The abnormalities demonstrated as the results of prolonged smoking, that is the chronic changes, may have mechanisms completely different from those which cause the evanescent and acute functional changes.

The rate at which pulmonary function declines in smokers as compared with non-smokers has been studied by Fletcher (5), by Higgins (6), and more recently by Comstock and associates (7). All agree on the finding of a decrease in forced expiratory volume

(FEV) and an increase in symptoms proportional to the extent of smoking; exsmokers showed improvement. It has also been reported by Massaro and associates (8) that the incidence of chronic obstructive lung disease in a hospitalized population of U. S. veterans was only 50% as high in the Negro as in the white. No racial differences were observed with respect to frequency or amount of smoking or type of tobacco smoked. Hayes (9) more recently reported a postmortem study of the lungs of native Jamaicans and was unable to demonstrate any difference in frequency or severity of panacinar emphysema between Negro, Chinese, East Indian, or Caucasians; nor any significant difference in "focal" emphysema in the larger Negro and small white groups. Hayes found no difference in the incidence of emphysema between rural and urban dwellers and suggested that other factors such as cigarette smoking may be responsible for the differences observed. Cederlof (10) and his associates studied the association between smoking and cardiovascular and respiratory symptoms. Genetic factors appeared to be of greater importance in the development of coronary symptoms than in respiratory. However, even the respiratory symptoms appeared to be influenced by genetic factors.

Cigarette smoking may induce its effect on the lung and bronchi by predisposing to intercurrent infections. Finklea and coworkers (11) performed a prospective study on 1,811 male college students. A higher incidence of illness was observed in the smokers of one pack or more daily, both by questionnaire and by an increased incidence of positive serologic titer for respiratory viral disease. The suggestion was made that subclinical illness occurred more frequently in the cigarette smoking population. This observation is supported by the experiments in mice by Spurgash and associates (12), who demonstrated increased susceptibility to aerosol challenges of K. pneumoniae and D. pneumoniae in cigarette smoke exposed animals. No decreased resistance was observed to PR-8 strain of type A influenza.

Acute inhalation of cigarette smoke decreased bronchial clearance of radioactive iron oxide particles in animals; in chronic human cigarette smokers the bronchial clearance also is usually impaired (13). Dalhamn and Rylander (14) demonstrated that a dose response relationship exists between acute inhalation of cigarette smoke constituents and ciliotoxicity, while the study of Pavia, Short and Thomson (15) failed to demonstrate any impaired clearance of radioactive particles administered by aerosol in chronic smokers as compared to non-smokers. These differences in findings relate more to studies in chronic smokers than to acute effects, and could well be due to factors other than the cigarette smoking. The studies of Green (16) have demonstrated that cigarette smoke interferes with phagocytic activity of alveolar macrophages. Such a mechanism could account for lowered resistance to infection and possibly for some effect on the prolonged phases of bronchial clearance.

One of the components of cigarette smoke which has received relatively little attention is cadmium. This material is of considerable interest since it has been reported that chronic occupational cadmium poisoning in man can induce pulmonary emphysema. It is also well recognized that cadmium is a common contaminant of polluted urban atmospheres. Hickey and his coworkers (17) consider that cadmium concentration is the best predictor of mortality from "diseases of the heart". Cadmium is present in cigarette smoke and is inhaled with the smoke (18). Considerable quantities of cadmium may thus be accumulated in the lungs of cigarette smokers over a period of years. This subject is worthy of considerably more investigation.***

Experimental studies attempting to produce either chronic bronchitis or emphysema in animals have been far from satisfying. Lamb and Reid (19) exposed rats to cigarette smoke from a Wright Autosmoker in differing doses over a period of 6 weeks. Exposures were performed 5 days a week, for periods up to 3.5 hours a day. The exposed animals failed to gain weight and demonstrated an increase in goblet cell number in the bronchial tree in proportion to the dose of cigarette smoke. Higher doses produced an increase in mitotic activity of the epithelial cells; some animals showed a change in mucin type within the cells from sialomucin to

---

*** See Chapter 4 in "Metallic Contaminants and Human Health", this Series. (Eds.)

sulfomucin. This study demonstrates a non-specific response of the respiratory tract epithelium which simulates that seen in animals after exposure to relatively high doses of SO_2. This reaction, while suggestive of certain changes of chronic bronchitis, does not fulfill all the criteria necessary since no bronchial gland hyperplasia or airways obstruction has been demonstrated. The most prolonged and extensive study of the effects of cigarette smoke inhalation in animals has recently been reported by Hammond et al. (20). These studies involved 97 beagles who smoked varying numbers of cigarettes through tracheostomy stomas for periods up to 876 days. Smoking dogs were reported to have a statistically significant incidence of emphysema. This study has evoked considerable comment and criticism and needs to be confirmed by additional studies.

Finally, the studies of Dontenwill (21) on hamsters exposed to cigarette smoke have demonstrated an increase in erythrocyte count after the 50th day of exposure, a decrease in food consumption and a decrease in skin temperature. Precancerous changes were seen in the larynx of most animals exposed for 10 months or more. Major abnormalities in the lung and trachea were not reported.

The inability to produce major abnormalities in the lung and trachea of experimental animals in these and other studies may be the result of differences in delivery of smoke, differences in species susceptibility or reaction, and a host of other factors, among which may be the necessity for exposure to additional etiologic or injurious agents. The need for multiple factors may thus be supported by the relatively negative results of experimental studies with cigarette smoke inhalation.

AIR POLLUTION AS ETIOLOGIC AGENT

The effects of ambient air pollution on the production of chronic obstructive lung disease are perhaps more difficult to evaluate than are those of cigarette smoking. The evidence that catastrophic episodes can produce increased mortality and morbidity is amply documented in the Donora (1948) and London (1952) episodes. Evidence is now substantial from the work of Greenberg (22), Cassal

(23) and others that moderate increases in air pollutant materials can likewise produce increases in morbidity, especially in individuals that have pre-existing pulmonary and cardiac disease. The interrelationships between air pollution and smoking are at times difficult to evaluate because of the overlays in these factors in may populations. However, it would appear the prevalence of respiratory symptoms and chronic obstructive lung disease, as determined epidemiologically, is linked to a high degree with cigarette smoking history. This has been ably documented by the study of Ferris (24), in which he compared the incidence of chronic obstructive lung disease in two populations, one exposed to moderate sources of air pollution and the other from a rural region. When these populations were compared in comparable age, sex, and smoking groups, there was a consistent excess in chronic obstructive lung disease at all age groups but one in the population from the polluted town. But the effect of smoking appeared far greater than that produced by the ambient pollution.

That atmospheric pollution alone can produce morbidity is seen best by studies in which infants and children of pre-smoking age are evaluated with regard to the concentration of pollutants present in their area of residence. The majority of these studies have been performed in Great Britain, but additional studies are available from the United States and other foreign nations to substantiate the observation that bronchitis and respiratory infections are seen with greater frequency in children who live in areas of heavier pollution. Toyoma and Tomona (25) studied the $FEV_{0.5}$ and FVC in 10 and 11 year old children and found that the measurements varied with the pollution index in "dirty" areas but not the clean ones. Douglas and Waller (26) studied the relationship of degree of air pollution to lower respiratory tract infection in children and observed a very real and significant correlation in both sexes regardless of social class. This was corroborated by the correlation of episodes of school absences with degree of pollution; here, however, there appeared to be a correlation with social class. A similar study has been reported by Lunn, Knowelden and Handyside (27) at Sheffield University. They demonstrated a relationship of level of atmospheric pollution of dwelling with the prevalence of upper and lower respiratory diseases and with impairment of $FEV._{75}$ and FVC in the area of most severe pollution. Ferris (28) in this country studied the relationship of level of air pollution and school absences in children of seven elementary schools of Berlin, New Hampshire. He found no significant differences between schools despite considerable differences in pollution levels. Chronic effects of air pollution are again more difficult to document because of the inter-play with associated etiological factors. The studies of Ishikawa et al. (29) indicate that in autopsy studies the incidence of anatomic emphysema is much greater in St. Louis, a city of considerably greater pollution than in Winnipeg. It is particularly important to observe that in non-smokers, more emphysema is observed in St. Louis than Winnipeg. When smokers were studied, there were four times the number of cases of severe emphysema in the more heavily polluted city. These findings are interpreted to indicate that smoking is not the only factor concerned with the development of emphysema and that a synergistic effect between smoking and environmental pollution may have occurred.

Experimental evidence concerning the effects of air pollution materials in the production of obstructive lung diseases is exceedingly difficult to interpret. This is due to the inadequate criteria which have been utilized for the evaluation of obstructive disease in exposed animals and because exposures have frequently been to single components of air pollutants. No effect on life span, weight, or histologic change in the lung was observed in rats exposed for their life span to Los Angeles atmospheric air (30). Similar results are reported by Vaughan and coauthors (31) who studied pulmonary function in 104 beagles exposed for 18 months to auto exhaust, NO_2 and SO_2. Amdur and her associates (32) studied the effects of sulfur dioxide in aerosols on the respiratory response of guinea pigs; and found that not all aerosols potentiate the SO_2 response, but several including NaCl, KCl, NH_4Cl and soluble salts of ferrous iron and other metals do. Lamb and Reid (33) have demonstrated that rats exposed to SO_2 by inhalation develop changes which they believe resemble chronic bronchitis in man. These changes

66

include goblet cell increase in airway epithelium, increase in mitotic activity of epithelial cells, increase in glycoprotein producing cells and increase in gland size. These changes persist for up to 5 weeks after exposure. Freeman and his associates (34) demonstrated a normal life span with persistent tachypnea in rats continuously exposed to 2 ppm NO_2. No changes in airflow resistance or dynamic compliance were observed. Histologically, the epithelium of the terminal airways showed a loss of exfoliative activity, a loss of cilia, and the appearance of intracytoplasmic crystalloid inclusions in the epithelial cells. They suggested that the cleansing function of the lung might be reduced. Numerous other studies have been performed which in general also have demonstrated that NO_2 in concentrations of 20-30 ppm, when utilized as a continuous exposure in hamsters, can produce only mild degrees of destructive emphysema. These experiments are not completely satisfying since they are created under circumstances which do not simulate the human exposure and in species which have a respiratory tract dissimilar in many respects from that of the human.

Reid (36) has lucidly and convincingly demonstrated that bronchitis in the young is frequently associated or correlated with factors other than the degree of urban air pollution. These factors are characterized as social and environmental conditions and include domestic overcrowding, increase in infections, and possibly dietary limitations. These observations again emphasize the interdependence of causative factors in the production of respiratory disease states, even in the relatively uncomplicated situation existing in children.

GENETIC FACTORS IN ETIOLOGY

A recent and exciting contribution to our understanding of some forms of chronic obstructive lung disease has been the observation of Laurell and Eriksson (37), amplified in the monograph by Eriksson (38). Their studies indicate that a marked deficiency of a serum factor migrating with the $alpha_1$ globulins is frequently associated with the presence of severe obstructive pulmonary disease in young individuals. This deficiency is transmitted as

a Mendelian autosomal trait and has been more
recently suggested to be transmitted as a codominant
trait. Clinically, the presence of the deficiency
can be detected in a number of ways: (1) by the
assay of serum for trypsin inhibitory capacity (TIC);
(2) by quantitative immunologic assay for the
specific protein alpha$_1$ - antitrypsin; (3) by
cellulose acetate electrophoresis; (4) by acid starch
gel electrophoresis; and (5) by antigen-antibody
crossed electrophoresis. The latter two methods are
sophisticated means for distinguishing true
heterozygotes from normals with borderline low
values, but more importantly for distinguishing the
phenotypic variants present in the populations.
Generally speaking, serum analysis is performed by
simple cellulose acetate electrophoresis; by serum
TIC assay supplemented by quantitative immunoassay.
A trimodal distribution is most frequently observed
of: (a) normals; (b) heterozygotes with intermediate
values approximately 50 - 60% of normal; and (c) a
severely deficient group, the homozygous deficiences
with levels of 5 - 20% of normal. The early studies
of Erikson suggested that the vast majority of
homozygous deficient persons suffered a severe degree
of chronic obstructive disease, which had an early
onset, progressed rapidly and was present with nearly
equal frequency in males and females. The disease
characteristics suggested severe emphysema rather
than bronchitis. Most subsequent reports have
confirmed this observation except for those of
Erkstan, Kiviloog and Ostlug (39) and Vidal et al.
(40), whose subjects demonstrated pronounced
bronchitis. Eriksson suggested that 1% of all cases
of chronic obstructive lung disease in Sweden was
likely to be associated with the severe alpha$_1$ -
antitrypsin deficiency, and he observed no increase
in incidences of chronic obstructive lung disease in
persons with heterozygous or intermediate deficiency
levels. If this were the case, this genetic form of
chronic obstructive lung disease would be little more
than an interesting curiosity, useful to confirm the
presence of hereditary factors and perhaps signal a
patho-genetic mechanism. Recently several groups in
this country have challenged the concept that
heterozygotes do not have a higher incidence of
chronic obstructive lung disease than control
populations. Lieberman's (41) studies of 66 patients
hospitalized with chronic obstructive lung disease

indicated that 25.8% have some form of the alpha$_1$ - antitrypsin deficiency, of which 15% are heterozygous. When patients under 50 years of age are considered, 48% demonstrated some deficiency. These findings have been confirmed by Kueppers, Fallat and Larson (42) in a group of 103 patients with chronic obstructive lung disease. These authors observed 5 homozygote deficients and 25 heterozygotes in this group, suggesting an increased occurrence of the obstructive lung lesions in heterozygotes. These findings are in contradiction to that reported by Welch and his associates (43), who found no relationship between intermediate levels of alpha$_1$ - antitrypsin deficiency and chronic obstructive lung disease. While no detailed smoking histories are available in these three groups of patients, Kueppers notes that 23 of his 25 heterozygotes were cigarette smokers, while in another publication from the Oklahoma group (Guenter et al. (44)), in which the patients with severe homozygous deficiency are described, it is noted that "those who smoked least appeared to have less severe disease or later onset of disease." Another factor of interest is that the two reports linking heterozygosity and chronic obstructive lung disease originate from large urban centers, where air pollution is severe, while the protagonist group derives their study from persons in a small urban center with considerably less pollution. Is it not possible that part or all of the deficiencies seen by these groups may arise from differences in ambient air pollution and smoking history? It may be of value to inquire if all persons with homozygous alpha$_1$ - antitrypsin deficiencies have chronic obstructive lung disease. These would probably be observed only in population studies. In the studies of Eriksson, 23 of the 33 closely examined cases of severe alpha$_1$ - antitrypsin deficiency had some form of chronic obstructive lung disease; Kueppers and associates claim that 90% of homozygous deficient persons who reach the age of 50 years have chronic obstructive lung disease. These studies both indicate that even homozygous deficiency is not necessarily associated with severe pulmonary abnormalities and again suggest that adjunct factors are needed. The age of onset of pulmonary disease in severe or homozygous deficiency is likewise of great interest. The reported cases as indicated above suggest that heavy smoking is often associated with early onset or more severe disease. In the reports of Levine et al. (45) three children ages 9, 12, and 14 are reported with the severe deficiency. None of these children demonstrated symptoms or abnormalities in standard pulmonary function tests; however, the oldest child demonstrated an abnormal pattern of distribution of pulmonary blood flow and increased dead space -- apparently the first evidence of the disease state. In the studies on children in which we are participating, non-specific respiratory disease states have been observed in children with heterozygous deficiency states, suggesting again an interplay of genetic and infectious factors even at this early age. Larson and his associates (46) have demonstrated a prevalence of abnormalities of pulmonary function among relatives of patients with chronic obstructive lung disease who do not have an alpha$_1$ - antitrypsin deficiency which was greater than that in a control group. This suggests that other genetic factors as yet unspecified may be of importance in the genesis of chronic obstructive lung disease. It is their feeling that heredity and smoking contribute equally to the likelihood of development of chronic obstructive lung disease.

OCCUPATIONAL FACTORS IN ETIOLOGY

The importance of occupational dust inhalation as a contributing factor in chronic obstructive lung disease has been debated since the inception of our industrial civilization. This subject has been more extensively studied by our British colleagues, and the major part of our information is derived from their studies. C. R. Lowe (47), Professor of Social and Occupational Medicine at the Welsh National School of Medicine, claimed that the differences in bronchitis death rates for miners and their wives, compared with agricultural workers and their wives, was due to occupation. Gilson (48), however, observed that the ratio of male to female death rate for bronchitis showed no clear relation to social class, although clearly the death rate from bronchitis (Table 1) was excessive in the miner.

He suggested that an alternative interpretation of the data might be "a multiplicative factor" nearly constant between the sexes, poorly related to occupation, and related mostly to socio-economic factors. National Morbidity studies in Great Britain

TABLE 1 -- BRONCHITIS STANDARDIZED DEATH RATE (Per million) 1949-53,
in males aged 16-64 (modified from Lowe 1969) (47)

	Social class							Certain occupations				
	I	II	III	IV	V	Differ-ence V-I	Ratio V/I	M	TW	AW	Differ-ence M-AW	Ratio M/AW
Males	160	249	461	475	804	644	5.0	733	465	263	470	2.8
Married females	35	49	101	123	154	119	4.4	167	94	91	76	1.9
Difference (M-F)	125	200	360	352	650		566	371	172			
Ratio M:F	4.6	3.2	4.6	3.9	5.2			4.4	5.0	2.9		

M, miners. TW, transport workers. AW, agricultural workers.

71

showed a pattern relating social class and occupations to absences for bronchitis (Table 2).

When morbidity from "all causes" and from bronchitis was analyzed and related to occupation, differences were apparent. Miners and quarrymen had the highest number of days of incapacity from all causes while the bronchitis rate was proportional to the morbidity from "all other causes". The bronchitis rate of the miners was not proportionately higher than the rate in engineers or construction workers, although it was a considerably higher proportion of all morbidity than that observed in clerical workers, agricultural workers, salesmen, and technical workers. The highest rate of bronchitis was observed in laborers (Table 3).

A large number of occupational field surveys have been performed in recent years to investigate the prevalence of bronchitis and respiratory symptoms in workers exposed to occupational factors. Gilson selected those studies which include the following pertinent data as adequate for analysis: high response rate, representative sampling of the population, use of standardized symptom questionnaire, measurement of FEV, and a record of smoking habits. The pattern observed is striking -- an excess of prevalence of respiratory symptoms and a lower ventilatory capacity in the dust-exposed groups compared with controls. The bronchitis prevalence ratio (exposed to controls) appears greater in cotton and flax workers. Other studies in this industry have been performed by Bouhuys and his associates (49) who reported an anomalous finding. In studies

TABLE 2 -- DAYS OF INCAPACITY FROM BONRCHITIS IN MALES AGED 18-63, AGE STANDARDIZED (Ministry of Pensions and National Insurance 1965) (Modified from (48))

Social Class	Days per 100 men	Social Class	Days per 100 men
All	123.5	IV:	
		Light	213.4
I and II	34.8	Medium	163.1
		Heavy	253.8 = 173.0
		Agricultural	46.8
III:			
Light	63.4		
Medium	100.1 = 95.4	V	265.1
Heavy	147.5		

TABLE 3 -- DAYS OF INCAPACITY FROM ALL CAUSES AND FROM BRONCHITIS, MALES AGED 18-63 AGE STANDARDIZED (Ministry of Pensions and National Insurance 1965) (Modified from (48))

Occupation	All causes	Bronchitis	Ratio of bronchitis to all causes
Miners and quarrymen	217	211	0.97
Coalface workers	199	154	0.76
Labourers (not exactly classified)	153	182	1.19
Drivers of stationary engines, cranes, etc.	125	141	1.13
Gas, coke, and chemical workers	116	131	1.13
Engineering and allied trades workers	99	101	1.02
Construction workers	99	105	1.06
Clerical workers	76	56	0.74
Agricultural workers	65	40	0.62
Sales workers	64	41	0.64
Professional and technical	55	33	0.60
Administrators and managers	39	16	0.41
All occupations	100	100	
Rate per 1,000 men	8,854	1,235	

of Spanish hemp workers, they observed that older (50-69 years) men with moderate to heavy smoking histories had significantly higher FEV_1 than non-smokers or light smokers. They interpreted this as indicating a self selection process involving the degree of response to hemp dust. Those workers who are smokers at age 50, are believed to be non-reactors, while the reactors by virtue of their symptoms become non- or ex-smokers at an earlier age. The general conclusion from these surveys is that bronchitis prevalence is increased about two-fold over controls. The part contributed by cigarette smoking in the increased prevalence of bronchitis in industry is no less difficult to evaluate here than in other situations. In the National Foundry survey in Great Britain in 1970, non-smokers had a lower prevalence of bronchitis in the control and foundry men; but the latter group had two times the rate of controls. Smoking increased the prevalence of bronchitis in both groups but tended to minimize the difference between them as the consumption of cigarettes increased. These findings differ from those reported by Sluis-Cremer (50) and associates, who studied the prevalence of bronchitis in mining and non-mining populations in South Africa. They found that chronic bronchitis was significantly more common in miners than in non-miners for every age and smoking category, with the exception of the non-smokers in whom no significant differences were observed in miners and non-miners.

The relationship of other factors such as duration of exposure, total dust load in the lung, and exposure to dust and fumes together on the prevalence of chronic bronchitis are less clear. No increased prevalence of bronchitis was noted in miners and ex-miners with increasing years at the coal face. On the other hand, men who worked on the foundry floor for increasing periods of time had a higher prevalence of bronchitis, even when corrected for cigarette smoking. Gilson has demonstrated quite clearly that there is no increase in prevalence of bronchitis with increasing category of simple pneumoconiosis; this suggests strongly that the total amount of dust in the lung with simple pneumoconiosis has no effect on the prevalence of bronchitis. This lack of correlation between simple pneumoconiosis and bronchitis may be explained if emphysema developed concurrently with the pneumoconiosis. That this may occur has recently been reported by Ryder and his associates (51). These investigators performed a correlated study of pathologic, radiologic, and physiologic findings in 247 coal miners and ex-miners and compared their findings to a control necropsy population matched for age and sex. Emphysema was much more commonly seen in the miners, both with simple and complicated pneumoconioses, than in the control population. The presence of this emphysema was best correlated with X-rays demonstrating the finer punctiform lesion by X-ray. Unfortunately, smoking histories are not presented in this study. While this report has several major flaws, its implications are of importance and should not be ignored without further study. Does the presence of coal dust in the lung predispose to disabling and destructive forms of emphysema? The implications of the recent experimental studies of Gross, Tuma and DeTreville (52,53) are not clear. This group reported that experimentally induced emphysema in hamsters imposed either prior to or following exposure to silicon dioxide or coal dust by inhalation or intratracheal inoculation, produced a decrease in the dust load of the lung when compared to controls. They attributed the decrease in residual lung dust to increase clearance.****

The preceding discussion indicates an increased morbidity and mortality from bronchitis in certain occupations which share the common factors of hard physical work, dust exposure at work, and adverse socio-economic factors. This excess bronchitis risk in dusty occupations is now about 2 or 3 times that in non-exposed groups. In any one subject, it is not possible to quantitate the several factors which may contribute to the presence of this occupational bronchitis or emphysema.

SUMMARY

The evidence for multiple factors participating in the etiology of chronic obstructive lung disease is reasonable. Each of these factors may however be considered as cofactor, rather than primary, since little is known of the initiating events and early or subclinical stages in the development and progression of these diseases. Pathologic studies of well-developed cases indicate that several forms of tissue alteration can exist and it is unlikely that a single agent or injury is responsible for the diverse pathologic changes. It is useful to recognize that cigarette smoke and air pollution are complex mixtures of gases, particulates and fumes, and combination of these agents may effect the anatomic and functional alterations, provided they are applied with sufficient frequency. There is no indication as to how these agents may cause tissue breakdown such as is seen in emphysema, although their effects in causing epithelial hyperplasias and metaplasias and glandular hyperplasias of chronic bronchitis are well documented. The intermediate for the induction of the destructive phase may be intercurrent viral or bacterial infection of the respiratory apparatus. Occupational exposures also may be considered as cofactors rather than primary or initiating events.

**** See also "Pulmonary Reactions to Coal Dust" in this Series. (Eds.)

75

Most studies suggest that prolonged and heavy cigarette smoking is of greater importance in producing chronic obstructive lung disease than either occupational or neighborhood air pollution exposures.

The genetic deficiency state of the serum protein alpha$_1$ antitrypsin, and its well documented relationship to chronic obstructive lung disease, has created considerable speculation regarding pathogenesis and progression of these disease entities. If it is true that only individuals with the homozygous or severe deficiency of the alpha$_1$ antiprotease have an increased susceptibility to chronic obstructive lung diseases, then the relatively small number of such individuals makes it unlikely that this factor plays an important part in the general nongenetic forms of this disease. The relative susceptibility of the heterozygote or intermediate deficiency form is still under study. The exact mechanism by which tissue destruction or emphysema follows the deficiency is not well understood, but an attractive suggestion is that leukocytic proteases released during intercurrent infection or inflammation may be inadequately neutralized by deficient serum antiproteases and injure surrounding tissues. This picture is mimicked experimentally by exposing animals to intratracheal aerosols of the proteolytic enzyme papain. Once again the deficiency state of the alpha$_1$ antiprotease may be considered as a necessary cofactor in the production of these disease states.

The complexities of considering etiology are obvious. Not one of the various factors discussed will necessarily produce the picture; combinations are strongest in producing the diseases. The intricate web of pathogenesis is at the present time insufficiently defined to evaluate the relative importance of each of the factors contributing to the etiology and the specific role that each may play.

REFERENCES

1. Prindle, R. A. et al. (1963). Comparison of pulmonary function and other parameters in two communities with widely different air pollution levels. Amer. J. Public Health 53: 200.

1a. Wright, G. W. Personal Communication.

2. Advisory Committee to the Surgeon General, PHS,
    DHEW. (1964). Report on Smoking and Health.
    PHS Publ. 1103. Govt. Print. Off.,
    Washington, D. C.

3. Nadel, J. A. and Comroe, J. H. (1961).
    Acute effects of inhalation of cigarette smoke
    on airway conductance. J. Appl. Physiol. 16:
    713.

4. Krumholz, R. A., Chevalier, R. B. and Ross,
    J. C. (1965). A comparison of pulmonary
    compliance in young smokers and non-smokers.
    Amer. Rev. Resp. Dis. 92: 102.

5. Fletcher, C. M. (1968). Bronchial infection
    and reactivity in chronic bronchitis. J. Roy.
    Coll. Phys., London 2: 183.

6. Higgins, I. T. et al. (1968). Chronic
    respiratory disease in an industrial town: A
    nine year follow-up study. Amer. J. Public
    Health 58: 1667.

7. Comstock, G. W. et al. (1970). Cigarette
    smoking and changes in respiratory findings.
    Arch. Env. Health 21: 50.

8. Massaro, D., Cuseck, A. and Katz, S. (1965).
    Racial differences in incidence of chronic
    bronchitis. Amer. Rev. Resp. Dis. 92: 94.

9. Hayes, J. A. (1970). Racial, occupational,
    and environmental factors in relation to
    emphysema in Jamaica. Chest 57: 136.

10. Cederlof, R., Friberg, L. and Hrubec, Z.
    (1969). Cardiovascular and respiratory symptoms
    in relation to tobacco smoking. Arch. Env.
    Health 8: 934.

11. Finklea, J. F., Sandifer, S. H. and Smith, D.
    D. (1969). Cigarette smoking and epidemic
    influenza. Amer. J. Epidemiol. 90: 390.

12. Spurgash, A., Ehrilich, R. and Petzold, R. (1968). Effect of cigarette smoking on resistance to respiratory infection. Arch. Env. Health 16: 385.

13. Albert, R. E., Lippmann, M. and Briscoe, W. (1969). The characteristics of bronchial clearance in humans and the effects of cigarette smoking. Arch. Env. Health 18: 738.

14. Dalhamn, T. and Rylander, R. (1968). Ciliotoxicity of cigarette smoke and its volatile components. Amer. Rev. Resp. Dis. 98: 509.

15. Pavia, D., Short, M. and Thomson, M. L. (1970). No demonstrable long-term effects of cigarette smoke on the mucociliary mechanism of the human lung. Nature 226: 1228.

16. Green, G. M. and Carolin, D. (1967). The depressant effect of cigarette smoke on the in-vitro anti-bacterial activity of alveolar macrophages. New Eng. J. Med. 276: 421.

17. Hickey, R. J., Schoff, E. P. and Clelland, R. C. (1967). Relationship between air pollution and certain chronic disease death rates. Arch. Env. Health 15: 728.

18. Nandi, M. et al. (1969). Cadmium content of cigarettes. Lancet 2: 1329.

19. Lamb, D. and Reid, L. (1969). Goblet cell increase in rat bronchial epithelium after exposure to cigarette and cigar tobacco smoke. Brit. Med. J. 1: 33.

20. Hammond, E. C. et al. (1970). Effects of cigarette smoking on dogs. Arch. Env. Health 21: 740.

21. Dontenwill, W. (1970). Experimental investigations on the effect of cigarette smoke inhalation on small laboratory animals. Inhalation Carcinogenesis, A.F.C. Symposium Series 18: 389.

22. Greenburg, L. et al. (1962). Report of an air pollution incident in New York City: November, 1953. Public Health Rpts. 77: 7.

23. Cassal, E. G. et al. (1965). Two acute air pollution episodes in New York City: Health effects. Arch. Env. Health 10: 364.

24. Ferris, B. (1968). Epidemiologic studies on air pollution and health. Arch. Env. Health 16: 541.

25. Toyama, T. and Tomona, Y. (1961). Pulmonary ventilatory capacity of school children in a heavily air polluted area. Jap. J. Public Health 8: 659.

26. Douglas, J. W., Bau, D. and Waller, R. E. (1966). Air pollution and respiratory infection in children. Brit. J. Prev. Soc. Med. 20: 1.

27. Lunn, J. E., Knowelden, J. and Handyside, A. J. (1967). Patterns of respiratory illness in Sheffield infant school children. Brit. J. Prev. Soc. Med. 21: 7.

28. Ferris, B. (1970). Effects of air pollution on school absences and differences in lung function in first and second graders in Berlin, New Hampshire, January 1966 to June 1967. Amer. Rev. Resp. Dis. 102: 591.

29. Ishikawa, S. et al. (1969). The emphysema profile in two midwestern cities in North America. Arch. Env. Health 18: 660.

30. Gardner, M. B. et al. (1969). Histopathologic findings in rats exposed to ambient and filtered air. Arch. Env. Health 19: 637.

31. Vaughan, T. R., Jennelbe, L. F. and Lewis, T. R. (1969). Long-term exposure to low levels of air pollutants. Arch. Env. Health 19: 45.

32. Amdur, M. O. and Underhill, D. (1968). The effects of various aerosols on the response of guinea pigs to SO_2. Arch. Env. Health 16: 460.

33. Lamb, D. and Reid, L. (1968). Mitotic rates, goblet cell increase and histochemical changes in mucus in rat bronchial epithelium during exposure to SO_2. J. Pathol. and Bacteriol. 96: 99.

34. Freeman, G. et al. (1968). Lesion of the lung in rats continuously exposed to 2 ppm NO_2. Arch. Env. Health 17: 181.

35. Kleinerman, J. (1971). Emphysema and bronchial epithelial hyperplasia in hamsters exposed to long-term NO_2. Amer. J. Pathol. 62: 93a.

36. Reid, D. D. (1969). The beginnings of bronchitis. Proc. Roy. Soc. Med. 62: 1.

37. Laurell, C. B. and Eriksson, S. (1963). The electrophoretic alpha one globulin pattern of serum in alpha one antitrypsin deficiency. Scand. J. Clin. Lab. Invest. 15: 132.

38. Eriksson, S. (1965). Studies in alpha one antitrypsin deficiency. Acta Med. Scand. 177: 175.

39. Erkstan, G., Kiviloog, G. J. and Ostlug, E. (1968). Alpha one antitrypsin deficiency and chronic pulmonary disease. Scand. J. Resp. Dis. 49: 311.

40. Vidal, J. et al. (1970). Deficits en alpha one antitrypsine, groupes Pi et broncho-pneumopathies chroniques. La Presse Medicale 78: 783.

41. Lieberman, J. (1969). Heterozygous and homozygous alpha one antitrypsin deficiency in patients with pulmonary emphysema. New Eng. J. Med. 281: 279.

42. Kueppers, F., Fallat, R. and Larson, R. K. (1969). Obstructive lung disease and alpha one antitrypsin deficiency gene heterozygosity. Science 165: 899.

43. Welch, M. T. et al. (1969). Antitrypsin deficiency in pulmonary disease: The significance of intermediate levels. Ann. Int. Med. 71: 533.

44. Guenter, C. A. et al. (1968). The pattern of lung disease associated with alpha one antitrypsin deficiency. Arch. Int. Med. 122: 254.

45. Levine, B. W. et al. (1970). Alteration in distribution of pulmonary blood flow. An early manifestation of alpha one antitrypsin deficiency. Ann. Int. Med. 73: 397.

46. Larson, R. K. et al. (1970). Genetic and environmental determinants of chronic obstructive pulmonary disease. Ann. Int. Med. 72: 627.

47. Lowe, C. R. (1969). Industrial bronchitis. Brit. Med. J. 1: 463.

48. Gilson, J. C. (1970). Occupational bronchitis. Proc. Roy. Soc. Med. 63: 857.

49. Bouhuys, A., Schilling, R. S. and van de Woestijne, K. P. (1969). Cigarette smoking, occupational dust exposure, and ventilatory capacity. Arch. Env. Health 19: 793.

50. Sluis-Cremer, G. K., Walters, L. G. and Sichel, H. S. (1967). Chronic bronchitis in miners and nonminers: An epidemiologic survey of a community in the gold mining area in the Transval. Brit. J. Indust. Med. 24: 1.

51. Ryder, R. et al. (1970). Emphysema in coal workers' pneumoconiosis. Brit. Med. J. 3: 481.

52. Gross, P. and DeTreville, R. T. P. (1969).
Emphysema and pneumoconiosis: An experimental
study on their interrelationship. Arch. Env.
Health 18: 340.

53. Gross, P., Tuma, J. and DeTreville, R. T. P.
(1971). Emphysema and Pneumoconiosis: A
comparative quantitation of dust content of
pneumoconiotic rodent lungs with and without
emphysema. Arch. Env. Health 22: 194.

CHAPTER 6. MULTIPLE FACTORS IN THE CAUSATION OF RENAL DISEASE

EDWARD H. Kass, Channing Laboratory,
Thorndike Memorial Laboratory, Harvard Medical School
and Boston City Hospital, Boston, Massachusetts

A discussion of multiple factors in the causation of environmentally induced disease of the kidneys carries with it several assumptions. First, of course, is that there are environmentally induced diseases of the kidneys, and of this there can be no doubt. The second is much more difficult to deal with, namely that when we discuss multiple factors, we imply that the interaction is meaningful in terms of ultimate prevention and perhaps even suggest that control based on any one factor may not be entirely or even significantly useful. For the latter statements to be acceptable, it would require study of such complex design that it appears unlikely that we shall in the near future be able to progress from articles of faith to statements based on meaningful data. We are all painfully aware that the multiple factor hypothesis is, at present, negative in content and is based more on the failure to identify single necessary (if not sufficient) causes of chronic disease than on the positive identification of the essential nature of the interaction of multiple factors. This absence of hard and meaningful data has seldom been a deterrent to the academic community. On the other hand, if ignorance of understanding of the best approaches to prevention of disease is a reasonable basis for stimulation of investigation, we cannot doubt that those who have undertaken to study the etiology of chronic disease merit a very high level of support.

I have divided the problems relating to the kidney into three general areas: toxic agents in the environment, the role of environment in infectious and immunological disease of the kidney, and finally, speculations concerning hypertension as an environmentally induced disorder of small children, perhaps operating through an effect on the kidneys.

ENVIRONMENTAL TOXINS AFFECTING THE KIDNEY

A number of heavy metals have been identified as causes of acute and/or chronic renal disease. Lead, cadmium, arsenic, mercury, copper, the heavy radioactive metals such as uranium, and many others have been implicated as causes of kidney disease, sometimes in consequence of industrial exposures and sometimes after other types of encounters with the heavy metals. Perhaps the best studied instance of nephropathy is that due to lead. Lead nephropathy is a special instance of the more general problem of lead poisoning, which occurs principally in small children who live in old houses that were once painted with paints containing lead. The children ingest the lead by gnawing at window sills or railings, or by picking up flakes of paint in their fingernails and chewing these. In the remarkable studies from Queensland, that are now quite classic, the high rate of lead poisoning in children was related to the architectural practice of building houses with open verandas surrounded by lead-painted railings. The children played on these verandas commonly and acquired lead by one of the several methods of ingestion. In the less spacious, crowded tenements, it has been observed that the children who gnaw at window sills or eat flakes of paint often have special behavioral characteristics, so that the problem of lead poisoning is compounded not only by the problem of antiquated housing, but also by specific psychological characteristics that seem particularly to predispose the child to the practice that results ultimately in lead poisoning. Perhaps it is the psychological characteristic that accounts for why the number of cases of lead poisoning, needlessly large as an absolute, is nevertheless very much smaller than would be expected from the numbers of children who have been raised in dwellings in which the use of lead paint was almost universal. Thus it becomes important to discuss prevention of lead poisoning in terms of removal of outdated housing, but perhaps this alone will not have much effect on the regressive behavior of the children. Similarly, it is of the utmost importance that children with lead poisoning be treated in a precisely defined manner, because lead which has been deposited in the bone is not very harmful, whereas when the lead has been mobilized from the bone, it may become harmful.

It is not my intent to discuss in detail the industrial exposures to lead and to other heavy metals. These are well-known and well-documented.* There has been much speculation that deposition of heavy metals in the kidneys at levels short of the frankly clinical may produce a situation which makes it easier for the kidney to be damaged by nephrotoxic or nephropathogenic agents, whether these be analgesics or bacteria. There is little evidence to support this possibility.

No discussion of nephropathies of unknown etiology can omit mention of the Balkan nephropathies. This group of diseases, perhaps this disease, has been identified principally in Rumania, Yugoslavia, and Bulgaria. It occurs in certain limited areas within these countries, with the areas characterized as being villages that are in the low-lying valleys, with adjacent valleys higher in the hills being relatively unaffected. The disease may have such high prevalence in endemic areas that it becomes the commonest cause of death, and as many as 75% of the households of some villages may be affected by progressive renal failure. The disease progresses insidiously and shows itself clinically as progressive renal failure, accompanied by relatively low levels of proteinuria with occasional accompanying hematuria, and in some regions, accompanying papilloma of the renal pelvis. Hypertension and edema are uncommon. Extensive studies of the water, soil, and tissues obtained from patients have failed to uncover any infectious or environmental agents that account for the disease. Extensive searches for trace elements and for heavy metals have shown a few unusual discoveries. It has been found that much slivovic (the popular plum

---

* See Metallic Contaminants and Human Health in this Series.

brandy) is unusually rich in copper because it is boiled in copper pots of a characteristic type, but this has been ruled out as a cause of the nephropathy. Lead has been found in one region because a mill had an excess concentration of lead in a material used to fill holes in the millstones. However, this was too localized to account for the distribution of the Balkan nephropathy. A variety of other studies have been conducted, too numerous to summarize at this time, but the syndrome remains a major mystery, and it is clearly environmental in origin, sparing those who have moved away from the affected regions if they move early enough in life, and afflicting some of those who have moved into the regions that are affected.

NEPHROTOXIC DRUGS

One of the causes of kidney disease that is eliciting increasing concern is that related to nephrotoxic antibiotics and other drugs. A wide variety of antimicrobial drugs are toxic to the kidneys to varying degrees. The evidence that they may cause chronic renal disease is less precise. There are, however, increasing concerns among clinicians that rates of renal failure are rising in hospitals, and there are indications that this rising rate may be related to the increasing use of toxic antibiotics. The precise mechanisms by which these drugs produce their effects are not yet clear, except in the case of the polypeptide antibiotics such as the polymyxins, in which there is strong evidence of direct binding by the acidic phospholipids of cell membrane. The degree to which individual differences and associated events in the kidney alter toxicity is just beginning to be understood. Since many of the toxic drugs are weak acids or weak bases, even as simple a variable as pH may affect the degree of toxicity, and since the pH of the urine is mostly controlled by diet, with high protein diets leading to the most acid urines, it is obvious that the dietary style of an individual or a group may influence substantially the relative toxicity of commonly used compounds. The list of renal toxic compounds that may be encountered in ordinary life is immense. Among those most often encountered clinically are the chlorinated hydrocarbons such as carbon tetrachloride and tetrachlorethylene, the short-chain alcohols such as methanol and the common glycols that are used as antifreezes, the commonly used analgesic drugs, and many others. No specifically useful purpose will be served at this time by listing each of these; such lists are readily available in the literature. It is of particular interest, however, that there have been claims of association between the effects of excessive ingestion of analgesics and bacterial infection, with some evidence that the analgesic-damaged kidney may be particularly susceptible to infection. The latter evidence is largely derived from studies in experimental animals and is at present being tested in a substantial epidemiological study in Switzerland; a final judgment must be kept in abeyance.

INFECTIOUS AND IMMUNOLOGICAL DISORDERS OF THE KIDNEY

The commonest infectious disorder affecting the kidney is, of course, bacterial pyelonephritis. Extensive studies of bacteriuria have shown only minor differences based upon different environmental and racial patterns, but there is still inadequate information concerning the relative rates of renal involvement in association with bacteriuria in different populations. Although a large number of environmental influences, including local trauma such as due to sexual activity, baths, direction of fecal cleansing with toilet tissue, and many other possibilities have been widely implicated as providing a basis for the appearances of infection, none of these has any body of evidence to support it. The most commonly held thesis, that infection of the urinary tract follows increased sexual activity, is difficult to accept in the face of overwhelming evidence that rates of bacteriuria rise in almost linear fashion by about 1% per decade in all females from age 5 to age 65. Acute post- streptococcal glomerulonephritis has not received as much epidemiological study as has rheumatic fever. Accordingly, some of the findings that are characteristic of a relationship between beta-hemolytic streptococci and acute rheumatic fever have not been adequately confirmed in the case of acute post-streptococcal glomerulonephritis. To this observer, one of the most critical findings in relation to rheumatic fever has been the observation that rates of rheumatic heart disease in a number of towns and cities in England varied directly with the numbers of persons per household. This concept has received recent support from the studies of Lilienfeld and his associates in Baltimore, who demonstrated that in upwardly mobile black families, rheumatic fever was still occurring despite the rise in socioeconomic indicators. The one variable that remained unaffected was the number of individuals per bedroom. It is, of course, reasonable to anticipate that pathogens that spread by contiguity, either through respiratory secretions, direct contact, or similar means that depend upon close association between individuals, would have their greatest effect when these individuals were thrust in close contact for an extended period of time, such as the overnight sleeping period. Speculations concerning the effect of size of inoculum, as a function of crowding, on the severity of infectious disease are supported by a certain number of observations that indicate that, for example, meningococcal meningitis, trachoma, and perhaps other infections are particularly likely to occur in relation to crowding within the household. These are difficult variables to separate from the other socioeconomic indicators, but some effective work in this direction has suggested that it may be worth examining, as a problem in social engineering, the cost of diluting the population by providing more ample household space as compared with the cost of the succession of acute and chronic illnesses that tend to cluster within a household, often on the basis of increased density of the individuals involved.

Recent indications that chronic glomerulonephritis may be related to the presence of certain viruses in the glomeruli, and the recent demonstration of an association between the nephropathy of disseminated lupus erythematosis and EB virus, raise the question of whether we are dealing exclusively with viral load, or whether individual immunological predispositions provide the basis for the chronic and usually progressive disease. Unfortunately, our knowledge of these interactions is rudimentary.

HYPERTENSION AS AN ACQUIRED DISORDER OF CHILDHOOD

Finally, I have the temerity to raise another set of multifactorial considerations, this time in relation to the possible etiology of hypertension. In brief, it has been recognized for more than a decade that the regression coefficient of blood pressure in adults, against the blood pressures of their first order relatives, is in the order of 0.3. This regression relationship, similar to that found for body stature in first order relatives, has suggested that hypertension is a multifactorial disorder with most of the input coming from environment rather than from a dominant gene. The latter conclusion has been a subject of much controversy, which will not be reviewed here. One aspect of the problem that recently became of interest to us has been to try to determine when the familial relationship first became manifest. An initial examination of the data collected by Miall and his associates for individuals aged 16 - 65 suggested, on the basis of relatively small numbers, that the familial relationship was about as strong for those aged 16 - 25 as for those aged 56 - 65. This suggests that the familial relationship between the blood pressure of an individual and those of his first order relatives could be detected before age 16. Recently, Zinner, Levy and I have examined the problem in children aged 2 - 14 and have found that the regression coefficients for the sib-sib comparisons of blood pressures in these age ranges were no different from those found among adults.

There is now a substantial body of evidence to indicate that each of us tends to follow a given blood pressure track throughout his adult life, at least. Those who have entered a given survey, with blood pressures falling in a given quintile, tend to remain in that quintile through extended follow-ups. It would thus be suggested that the tracking phenomenon may be already established by early childhood. Just how early remains to be discerned in future observations. If one may put together what is now known about the epidemiology of hypertension, a speculative picture can be constructed.

The factor or factors responsible for the development of hypertension appear either in utero or during the first two years of life. These factors are almost universally present, but in many populations are seen more frequently in rural than in urban communities, and are more readily operative among the lower than the higher socioeconomic levels. The factors are readily shared by members of the family and there may be some genetic predisposition that helps to account for this sharing. Thus, in our search for the factor or factors that are etiologically significant, it may be of the utmost importance not to look at those who are middle-aged or older, but rather to look at the earliest years of life. Perhaps our inadequate understanding of the etiology of hypertension is related to our having searched for etiological factors some 40 or 50 years too late. Finally, in the same speculative mood, an argument may be presented to support the hypothesis that the major factors accounting for the familial distribution of blood pressure are not genetic. The argument hinges upon the finding, now widely confirmed, that there is a crude inverse relationship between fecundity and levels of blood pressure, and that this relationship is found in both sexes. Thus, the highest levels of blood pressure are associated with the fewest numbers of children. On this basis, hypertensives would appear to be at a net reproductive disadvantage. Thus, the disease is likely to be bred out of existence, and the fact that it is still with us must be argued on the basis of three possibilities. The first is that hypertension is a new disease and has not had time to breed itself out of existence in accordance with the lowered fecundity of hypertensives. This argument cannot be met squarely, but the fact that strokes are well described in the ancient writings suggests that hypertension is not a new disease. Secondly, hypertensives may enjoy a balanced polymorphism, which would help overcome the net reproductive disadvantage that accompanies the hypertensive state. Unfortunately, no evidence for such polymorphism has yet appeared and there is no indication that hypertensives tend to breed earlier or in some other way overcome the reproductive disadvantage that accompanies their state. The most likely alternative, therefore, is the third possibility, which is that hypertension is a familial acquired disorder in which the etiological factor or factors are passed through the environment, thus accounting for the familial tendency. As we have indicated earlier, this acquisition presumably occurs in the earliest stages of development of the individual, and perhaps that is the direction of search in which both environmentalists and those interested in hypertension should expend some of their efforts.

PART II

MECHANISMS OF MULTIFACTOR EFFECT

Here contributors were asked to go towards the other end of the spectrum and discuss how certain environmental factors may operate in combination to produce disturbances of function, and to describe the mechanisms involved. As knowledge progresses, the alternative approaches of Parts I and II will meet to produce a much clearer picture of environmentally induced disease in general. There are indications that this is already happening.

CHAPTER 7. INTERACTIONS OF CHEMICALS AS A RESULT OF ENZYME INHIBITION

KENNETH P. DUBOIS, Toxicity Laboratory,
University of Chicago, Chicago, Illinois

The problem of detecting interactions from exposure to combinations of chemical agents is one of the most complex tasks that the biologist has encountered because of the enormous number of chemicals and combinations to which exposures may occur.

For many years the conventional procedure for evaluating the toxicity of drugs, pesticides, and other chemicals has involved thorough acute and chronic toxicity tests on common laboratory animals. The scope of these toxicity tests has increased in recent years to include more species, measurements of age and sex differences in susceptibility, and possible adverse effects of chemicals on reproduction. The conventional toxicity studies usually provide the important basic information needed for establishing conditions for the safe use of a chemical agent for whatever purpose it is intended. The knowledge of the pharmacological actions of chemical agents that is gained during the conventional toxicity tests is used extensively to predict the type of response that would be expected from simultaneous exposure to combinations having the same or different pharmacological actions.

In the area of therapeutic agents a great deal of attention has been given over the years to prediction of the type of response to be expected from various drug combinations on the basis of general pharmacological actions. Additive effects are expected with two drugs producing similar changes in some organ system, and antagonistic actions are predictable by the same approach. Similarly, pesticidal chemicals belonging to the same chemical class generally have additive injurious effects that are predictable on the basis of a common mode of action. However, exceptions are sometimes noted in that the biological activity of combinations of drugs or combinations of pesticides is significantly greater or less than would be expected from their individual toxicities or their separate pharmacological actions. The extent to which this type of interaction may occur between combinations of pesticides, drugs, and environmental chemicals is a question of considerable concern.

The limited attention that has been given to interactions that alter the toxicity of chemicals has been focused largely on drugs. One reason for this is that it is entirely feasible to examine a limited number of combinations of drugs for interactions when it is known which drugs are likely to be given simultaneously or sequentially. In contrast, the search for interactions between drugs and the numerous occupational or environmental chemicals to which man may be exposed is far more difficult from the standpoint of the number of chemicals or even the number of different types of chemical classes of compounds that may be involved in interactions. A second important factor in limiting progress with regard to interactions involving environmental chemicals is that investigators competent to engage in research in this area tend to place a higher priority on drugs than on other chemicals.

To the extent that deviations from the expected responses for combinations of chemicals have been explained, it has frequently been found that one agent inhibits or stimulates the metabolism of the other compound. Thus it is reasonable to focus a great deal of attention on this mechanism, although it is well recognized that interactions can involve a number of other mechanisms.

The discovery (1-3) of the ability of chlorinated hydrocarbons to cause interactions through induction of hepatic microsomal enzymes has served as an outstanding example of the manner in which environmental chemicals can influence disease processes by changing the potency and effectiveness of drugs used to treat diseases. Prior to that discovery, essentially no attention was given to the possibility that this important class of pesticides would produce any effect, except possible additive actions acutely in combination with chemicals acting on the nervous system, or additive injury chronically in combination with other liver toxicants.

It is not the intention of this presentation to discuss the implications of enzyme induction by pesticides or any other chemicals as a cause of interactions, but it seems important in consideration of the whole subject to emphasize that the two major classes of insecticides, the chlorinated hydrocarbons and the organophosphates, which have been in use for the past 25 years, are both capable of causing interactions by different mechanisms that were recognized and explained through a biochemical mechanistic approach. The question that is largely unanswered is, how many other groups of environmental chemicals that have not been studied as thoroughly as the pesticides are capable of causing interactions? It is impractical to test all of the various combinations of chemicals to which man may be exposed, using toxicity or pharmacological responses as a guide. Advances in drug metabolism involving hepatic microsomal enzymes has made it possible to examine classes of chemical agents for inhibition or induction of these enzymes, and then to reliably predict the influence of alteration of the activity of microsomal enzymes on the toxicity of other chemicals. This presentation will attempt to illustrate again the usefulness of the biochemical approach to interactions, using the inhibitory action of the organophosphates on esterases as a practical example.

POTENTIATION OF MALATHION

The initial interest in interactions caused by pesticides was stimulated by Frawley et al. (4) in 1957, who found that marked potentiation of the toxicity of malathion results from simultaneous administration of another organophosphate, EPN, (O-p-nitrophenyl phenylphosphonothioate). (Potentiation of toxicity is indicated by a response which greatly exceeds that expected from the simple additive effect of two chemicals having the same mode of action). This observation was of special interest because knowledge of the pharmacological actions of pesticides obtained by conventional toxicity tests has always been used to predict the type of response that would be expected from simultaneous exposure to combinations of pesticides. Simple additive toxicity is the expected result from exposure to combinations of pesticides with anticholinesterase activity. The observation of potentiation of toxicity by a combination of EPN and malathion quickly led to the introduction of a requirement by the Food and Drug Administration that all new pesticides of the anticholinesterase class be tested in combination with each pesticide of this class for which tolerances had already been established, to determine whether potentiation of toxicity occurred. The usual procedure for obtaining this information has been measurement of the toxicity of combinations of the new anticholinesterase agent with each one of the existing compounds. As the number of anticholinesterase insecticides increased, the toxicity measurements required to ascertain whether any combinations cause potentiation of toxicity has become rather extensive. In addition, it has become apparent that the simultaneous administration of two compounds may not reveal the capability of one agent to potentiate the toxicity of the other compound. The importance of varying the time of administration of one agent with respect to the other one was clearly demonstrated by Hagan et al. (5) who found that the administration of Delnav (technical dioxathion containing 70% cis and trans isomer of 2,3-dioxane S,S=bis[0,0-diethyl phosphorodithioate]) four hours before malathion caused a much higher degree of potentiation than was observed following simultaneous administration of the compounds. In addition to these limitations to the use of acute toxicity tests for detecting interactions of this type, the number of toxicity measurements involved necessarily restricted the studies to a single species, which was usually the rat.

Within a relatively short time after the potentiation of toxicity of malathion by EPN was observed, the mechanism responsible for this effect

was explained (6,7) by observations that EPN inhibits
the enzymatic hydrolysis of the carboxyester linkages
of malathion. The hydrolysis of malathion is
catalyzed by one or more non-specific esterases,
called aliesterases. A parallel mechanism has been
shown (8) to be responsible for the potentiation by
EPN of the toxicity of dimethoate.

INHIBITION OF ALIESTERASES

As soon as the biochemical mechanism responsible
for the potentiation of the toxicity of malathion by
EPN was elucidated, it was clear to us (9) that more
attention should be given to a study of the metabolic
pathways involved in the detoxification of chemical
agents, with the understanding that food additives,
pesticides, and therapeutic agents containing similar
groups and linkages can be expected to utilize common
detoxification pathways. It thus seemed more logical
to approach the problem of interactions caused by
organophosphates as a result of inhibition of
aliesterases, by determining the no-effect
dietary levels for aliesterase inhibition for each
compound, instead of measuring the toxicity of
combinations of these compounds. Studies on
the biochemical mechanism of potentiation of
the toxicity of organophosphates made it
apparent that only one aspect of the implications
of aliesterase inhibition had been considered. Any
compound such as EPN which is capable of
inhibiting aliesterases would be expected to
inhibit, not only the detoxification of another
organophosphate, but also the hydrolytic
detoxification of any drug or other type of chemical
agent that is normally detoxified by aliesterases.
The process of testing the toxicity of various
combinations of organophosphates is too
restricted, even though it involves a large number of
toxicity tests.

To ascertain the ability of organophosphates to
potentiate the toxicity of other organophosphates and
other esters, it seemed logical to develop
biochemical methods that would quantitatively measure
the amount of inhibition of the non-specific
esterases and amidases that catalyze the
detoxification of foreign esters. It seems pertinent
to this discussion to indicate that the ability of
organophosphate insecticides to inhibit a number of

99

esterases has been known for more than 25 years, but that it was only within the last 10 years that the significance of this inhibition in relation to interactions was recognized. This illustrates the fact that essentially no thought had been given over the years to the influence of one environmental chemical on the toxicity of another one. The physiological importance of non-specific esterases in normal metabolism has not been clarified and, as a result, inhibition of their activity has been considered to be unimportant.

A quantitative procedure was developed (10) for measuring the inhibitory potency of organophosphate insecticides on aliesterases, using diethylsuccinate and tributyrin as substrates for carboxyesterases and acentanilid as a substrate for amidases. The high susceptibility of the enzyme that hydrolyzes tributyrin to inhibition by organophosphates had been well established in 1953 by Myers and Mendel (11). Diethylsuccinate is the portion of the malathion molecule that is detoxified by carboxylesterases and its high susceptibility to inhibition by the organophosphate, EPN, was well established from the potentiation studies which initially revealed this type of interaction (4,6,7).

When rats were fed various levels of EPN in the diet for 13 weeks, it was found that maximum inhibition of aliesterases and amidase occurred within one week after feeding the organophosphates was begun. Dose-related amounts of inhibition of diethylsuccinate and tributyrin hydrolysis were observed with dietary levels from 1 ppm to 25 ppm. The amidase that hydrolyzes acentanilid was somewhat less sensitive, in that a dietary level of 5 ppm was required to produce appreciable inhibition of this enzyme. The important consideration in connection with the practical significance of aliesterase inhibition is the relative susceptibility of cholinesterase and aliesterases. The aliesterases must be inhibited at levels well below those that produce cholinesterase inhibition to be of significance with regard to potentiation of the toxicity of various drugs and other chemicals containing ester linkages, because the permitted levels in food are always below the level that causes significant cholinesterase inhibition. The level of

EPN that produces inhibition of cholinesterase is above 5 ppm, thus indicating a greater susceptibility of aliesterases and amidase to inhibition.

More recent studies have shown (12) that nearly all of the common organophosphate insecticides are more effective inhibitors of aliesterases than of cholinesterase and are, therefore, capable of causing interactions at dietary levels that produce no toxic effects or inhibition of cholinesterase. There are marked differences in the susceptibility of the various aliesterases to organophosphates. Table 1 shows the dietary levels of several organophosphates that produce 50% inhibition of aliesterases and cholinesterase. Some insecticides such as Folex, ethion, and Ronnel exhibit exceedingly high potency as aliesterase inhibitors and low anticholinesterase activity.

Triorthotolyl phosphate (TOTP) is a potent inhibitor of aliesterases (Table 1), but it is a weak cholinesterase inhibitor and has low acute toxicity. While TOTP is not an insecticide, it is an important environmental chemical because of its various industrial uses. TOTP is used as a plasticizer in vinyl plastics manufacture, as an additive to extreme pressure lubricants, as a non-flammable fluid in hydraulic systems, and

TABLE 1 -- DIETARY LEVELS OF ORGANOPHOSPHATE INSECTICIDE COMPOUNDS THAT PRODUCE 50% INHIBITION OF ALIESTERASE ACTIVITY

| | Dietary level (ppm) for 50% inhibition | | | |
| Organo-phosphate | Diethylsuccinate hydrolysis | | Tributyrin hydrolysis | |
	Liver	Serum	Liver	Serum
Parathion	3.4	7.6	1.8	7.0
Methyl parathion	7.0	>25.0	2.3	>25.0
Systox	2.6	12.0	0.7	13.0
Di-Syston	2.1	8.5	0.6	9.0
Phosdrin	10.5	35.0	3.1	30.0
Guthion	25.1	102.0	10.0	>100.0
Trithion	3.4	7.6	0.4	6.0
Folex	1.0	3.7	3.1	3.9
Ethion	14.0	>25.0	0.9	>25.0
Malathion	270.0	>500.0	240.0	>500.0
Ronnel	21.0	40.0	8.0	37.0
Triorthotolyl phosphate	7.0	17.0	22.0	21.0

101

as a lead scavenger in gasoline. Thus, there are numerous possibilities for exposure to this compound. Over the years there have been periodic outbreaks of serious poisoning from the misuse of materials such as lubricant oils containing TOTP. Attention was always focused primarily on the demyelination that is a characteristic effect of high doses of this compound. No attention has ever been given to the aliesterase inhibition that must have occurred in all people exposed to appreciable amounts of this chemical. No surveys have ever been conducted on people occupationally exposed to TOTP to ascertain whether their ability to detoxify ester-type drugs is impaired.

The biochemical approach to the study of potentiation of toxicity through aliesterase inhibition represents a practical method of determining the dietary levels that might potentiate the toxicity of other insecticides, or other pharmacologically active compounds whose normal detoxification depends upon esterases.

The amount of inhibition of aliesterases that is required to produce a significant or substantial increase in toxicity of various esters is of importance in judging the significance of aliesterase inhibition. Information relating inhibition of aliesterases and potentiation of malathion toxicity was obtained by producing various levels of aliesterase inhibition. The same type of comparison could have been made using drugs such as local anesthetics, whose detoxification depends upon esterases. To obtain information on the amount of inhibition required to potentiate the toxicity of malathion, different dietary levels of EPN, parathion, Guthion, Folex, and TOTP were fed in the diet to rats for one week. The acute LD_{50} of malathion to these animals was then measured. Table 2 shows the amount of inhibition of aliesterase activity, and the amount of increase in the acute toxicity of malathion, in rats fed various levels of the organophosphates for one week.

These measurements showed that all of the compounds have the ability to inhibit aliesterases, and when the aliesterase activity is sufficiently decreased prior to administration of malathion the toxicity of this compound is increased. The dietary

TABLE 2 -- RELATIONSHIP BETWEEN POTENTIATION OF THE ACUTE TOXICITY OF MALATHION BY ORGANIC PHOSPHATES AND INHIBITION OF THE ENZYMATIC HYDROLYSIS OF DIETHYLSUCCINATE AND TRIBUTYRIN

Compound	Dietary Level (ppm)	Malathion LD$_{50}$ ± S.E. (mg/kg)	% of Normal Activity in Liver	
			Diethylsuccinate	Tributyrin
Control	0	600.5 ± 19.7	100.0	100.0
EPN	5	524.8 ± 25.8	68.2	47.1
	7	397.4 ± 23.7	35.6	23.7
	10	253.0 ± 14.9	16.6	11.3
Parathion	2	502.4 ± 40.7	61.3	29.3
	5	440.7 ± 27.3	28.6	14.7
TOTP	5	496.5 ± 10.8	62.8	77.6
	25	186.4 ± 23.1	14.5	44.3
	50	41.3 ± 4.3	5.4	18.3
Folex	1	569.5 ± 21.2	61.8	62.5
	5	303.5 ± 11.4	23.8	28.9
	15	46.0 ± 6.3	2.7	5.3
Guthion	5	562.9 ± 31.1	90.0	62.2
	25	525.0 ± 16.5	44.7	36.6

levels of each compound selected for these
measurements did not produce inhibition of the
cholinesterase activity of serum, brain, or liver.
Thus additive cholinesterase inhibition did not
contribute to the increased toxicity of malathion.

COMMENTS

Inhibition of detoxification enzymes by
environmental chemicals can set the stage for
interactions when subsequent exposure occurs to
another chemical agent, whose detoxification
depends upon a particular enzyme system. One manner
in which environmental chemicals can
interfere with detoxification is illustrated
by the inhibitory action of organophosphate
insecticides on aliesterases that catalyze the
hydrolysis of many exogenous chemicals containing
ester linkages. Toxic action of these
insecticides due to cholinesterase inhibition has
long been known, and all of the safety standards for
the use of these compounds have been based on
establishment of levels that will not inhibit
cholinesterase. It has also been known for many
years that the organophosphate insecticides
inhibit many non-specific esterases. However,
inhibition of non-specific esterases by a single
chemical agent causes no known physiological
disturbance or morphological changes. It is only
when the animal is subjected to a second chemical
whose detoxification is inhibited that the importance
of inhibition of aliesterases is seen. Until
recently very little attention has been given to the
importance of guarding against interactions of this
type in setting the permissible limits for food
additives, pesticides, and environmental chemicals.

A major difficulty in taking practical steps to
reduce the possibility of toxic interactions is the
vast number of combinations of chemical agents that
have to be considered. It is impractical to conduct
toxicity tests on all of the various combinations of
importance. However, in connection with inhibition
or stimulation of detoxification systems, biochemical
approaches are being developed which are eliminating
the necessity of conducting toxicity tests on vast
numbers of combinations of chemicals. It was the
attempt of this presentation to show that
quantitative measurements of the effects of esterase

inhibitors allow the establishment of permitted use levels of an organophosphate below the level that would inhibit the hydrolytic detoxification of any drug or chemical agent. By the use of this biochemical approach it is unnecessary to test numerous pairs of compounds to ascertain whether potentiation of toxicity occurs.

Biochemical procedures for the measurement of enzyme induction have already been well established. By the use of these procedures it is possible to ascertain which classes of environmental chemicals produce this effect and the dose-response relationships. Examination of the effects of important individual environmental chemicals and classes of chemicals on detoxification reactions should become a part of their routine toxicological evaluation. If this is done reasonable predictions can be made about interactions between various combinations of chemical compounds. The intensive study of drug metabolism reactions, and factors that affect these reactions, which has been conducted during the past decade has established important background information for a logical approach in the future to those interactions that involve detoxification processes.

SUMMARY

Chemical agents are among the multiple factors that may be involved as a cause of diseases or in the prolongation or exaggeration of disease processes. One mechanism by which chemicals can produce such effects is through interactions in which one chemical agent interferes with the metabolism of body constituents such as steroids, or with the metabolism of a second exogenous chemical. Interactions at the level of metabolism can occur from inhibition or stimulation of the activity of drug metabolizing enzymes. One example of this type of interaction has been demonstrated with organophosphate insecticides. These insecticides inhibit a number of non-specific esterases (aliesterases) in addition to their inhibitory effect on cholinesterase. Non-specific esterases play an important role in the detoxification of drugs and other chemicals containing ester linkages. Thus inhibition of non-specific esterases may result in potentiation of the toxicity of a variety of chemical agents. Doses of the organophosphates within the range to which occupational exposure may occur will inhibit aliesterases more effectively than cholinesterase. Thus an inability to detoxify chemicals by hydrolysis can occur with exposures to organophosphorus insecticides that are too low to cause any adverse effect that can be directly attributed to these pesticides. This type of interaction has received little attention in previous studies on people exposed to these insecticides but it should be included in future studies on the effects of low-level exposure to insecticides of the organophosphate class.

REFERENCES

1. Hart, L. G. and Fouts, J. R. (1963). Effects of acute and chronic DDT administration on hepatic microsomal drug metabolism in the rat. Proc. Soc. Exptl. Biol. Med. 114: 388.

2. Hart, L. G. and Fouts, J. R. (1965). Further studies on the stimulation of hepatic microsomal drug metabolizing enzymes by DDT and its analogs. Arch. Exptl. Pathol. Pharmakol. 249: 486.

3. Hart, L. G., Shultice, R. W. and Fouts, J. R. (1963). Stimulatory effects of chlordane on hepatic microsomal drug metabolism in the rat. Toxicol. Appl. Pharmacol. 5: 371.

4. Frawley, J. P. et al. (1957). Marked potentiation in mammalian toxicity from simultaneous administration of two anticholinesterase compounds. J. Pharmacol. Exptl. Therap. 121: 96.

5. Hagan, E. C., Jenner, R. M. and Fitzhugh, O. G. (1961). Acute toxicity and potentiation studies with anticholinesterase compounds. Fed. Proc. 20: 432.

6. Murphy, S. D. and DuBois, K. P. (1957). Quantitative measurement of inhibition of the enzymatic detoxification of malathion by EPN (ethyl p-nitrophenyl thionobenzene-phosphonate). Proc. Soc. Exptl. Biol. Med. 96: 813.

7. Cook, J. W. et al. (1958). Malathionase. I. Activity and inhibition. J. Off. Agr. Chemists 41: 399.

8. Uchida, T. and O'Brien, R. D. (1967). Dimethoate degradation by human liver and its significance for acute toxicity. Toxicol. Appl. Pharmacol. 10: 89.

9. DuBois, K. P. (1958). Potentiation of the toxicity of insecticidal organic phosphates. Amer. Med. Assoc. Arch. Env. Health 18: 488.

10. DuBois, K. P., Kinoshita, F. K. and Frawley, J. P. Quantitative measurement of inhibition of aliesterases, acylamidase, and cholinesterase by EPN and Delnav. Toxicol. Appl. Pharmacol. 12: 273.

11. Myers, D. K. and Mendel, B. (1953). Studies on aliesterases and other lipid-hydrolyzing enzymes. I. Inhibition of the esterases and acetoacetate production of liver. Biochem. J. 53: 16.

12. Su, M. et al. (1971). Comparative inhibition of aliesterases and cholinesterase in rats fed eighteen organophosphorus insecticides. Toxicol. Appl. Pharmacol. 20: 241.

CHAPTER 8. INTERACTIONS OF CHEMICALS AND DRUGS TO PRODUCE EFFECTS ON ORGAN FUNCTION

JAMES R. FOUTS, National Institute of Environmental Health Sciences, Research Triangle Park, North Carolina

First it is important to understand what I am and am not going to do in this paper. I wish to present a number of examples of how various chemicals can interact to produce effects on organ function not seen when exposure is to only one component of the mixture. These examples, while numerous, will be concerned primarily with a final effect thought to be mediated by actions of the chemicals on systems in liver microsomes. These hepatic microsomal enzymes are responsible for the metabolism of a variety of usually lipid soluble materials, both xenobiotics and natural, endogenous substances such as steroid hormones. I am not going to adequately cover the general area of drug and chemical interaction; this can involve sites of interaction in a variety of non-hepatic tissues and by mechanisms which include changing absorption, distribution, and excretion of the chemicals or their interactions with the "receptor site" whatever that is. These are all equally valid areas of concern and undoubtedly should be worried about more extensively in any comprehensive consideration of interactions.

The absorption, distribution, and excretion of a drug or chemical, as well as its interaction with receptor sites, can all be affected by its metabolism. Many of the processes involved in these aspects of drug or chemical disposition are affected by the chemical and physical properties of the drug or chemical, which can in turn be changed when that drug or chemical is metabolized.

Thus, lipid solubility of a drug or chemical has important effects on its absorption, distribution, excretion, metabolism, and interaction with receptors. Lipid solubility is markedly changed by most mechanisms of metabolism of drugs or chemicals. Many drug or chemical metabolites are totally different in all aspects of their disposition and receptor activity from the parent drug or chemical.

With these general remarks as an introduction, I would like to turn to some studies of interactions based on changing xenobiotic or steroid metabolism due to prior exposure to drugs or chemicals. Xenobiotic or steroid metabolism can be enhanced or slowed or both by prior exposure to drugs or chemicals. The ability of one chemical to affect the metabolism of itself and of other chemicals has been widely studied in pharmacology. Classic examples of these interactions include: (1) the inhibition of cholinesterases by organophosphorous insecticides and "nerve gases"; (2) the inhibition of monoamine oxidases by hydrazides; (3) the inhibition of drug-metabolizing enzymes in liver microsomes by a variety of drugs and chemicals; and (4) the stimulation of drug-metabolizing enzymes in liver microsomes by a variety of drugs and chemicals such as chlorinated insecticides, phenobarbital, and polycyclic hydrocarbons like benzpyrene. In the case of hepatic microsomal drug-metabolizing enzymes, inhibition of these enzymes is often followed by a phase of enzyme stimulation or induction -- the net effect on these enzymes will then depend on dose of inhibitor-stimulator, frequency of dosing, and interval between last dose of inhibitor-stimulator and assay of effect.

A major concern of this paper will be to present examples of interactions wherein at least one of the interacting components (factors, chemicals) is "environmental." There are many pitfalls in trying to define whether something is "environmental" and I do not care to engage in such polemics. I hope my examples will be acceptable and I will try to present those that I think will be interesting and relatively non-controversial. My own research has concerned how insecticides of the chlorinated hydrocarbon class can affect the hepatic microsomal metabolism of other

110

chemicals and drugs. In order to be clear about some of the things to be discussed, it is important to mention one other point -- the metabolism of a chemical or drug by enzymes like those of liver microsomes may produce metabolites that are more active, as well as those less active than the parent drug or chemical. Thus, speeding up the metabolism of the chemical may make it more or less toxic (active), depending on whether the metabolite is more or less active than the parent compound, and on whether the further metabolism of the metabolite is also speeded up. These considerations must not be forgotten in an enthusiastic rush to generalities. Drug and chemical interactions are often confusing enough without the limitations of an overgeneralized hypothesis to lead us astray.

Our studies on the effects of various organochlorine insecticides on hepatic microsomal enzymes in various animal species began in 1960. Much of the work is cited in two recent reviews (1, 2). The essence of our results suggests that a number of these insecticides (e.g., DDT and derivatives, chlordane and congeners) can be potent inducers (stimulators) of xenobiotic metabolism by hepatic microsomes in a variety of animal species including rats, rabbits, squirrel monkeys, and mice. Immediately after the dosing with these insecticides, an inhibition of these same enzymes may occur. The extent of this inhibition, its duration, and the enzymes affected depend on dose of the chlorinated insecticide, the route of its administration, the animal species studied, and the xenobiotic whose metabolism is affected; but the principle is common -- first, inhibition; then, stimulation (induction) of microsomal enzyme activity. Accompanying these effects of chlorinated insecticides on xenobiotic metabolism can be other actions on the liver. Most organochlorine insecticides cause increases in liver weight, increase in liver cell size and proliferation of the smooth endoplasmic reticulum (SER) of the hepatocyte. If exposure to insecticide continues for some time, the proliferated SER may consolidate to form whorls or fingerprints of concentric and tightly packed membranes; this state may have different implications for hepatotoxicity than acute proliferation of SER (3).

111

Certain liver functions besides xenobiotic metabolism (by microsomes) may be affected by exposure to insecticides like DDT or chlordane. Most of these have not yet been studied and we can only make certain predictions by analogy with other chemicals (like phenobarbital) which seem to produce effects on the liver similar to those seen after DDT or chlordane. The liver cell, after DDT or chlordane, is packed with new SER. Such SER could serve as a marked storage site for lipid-soluble materials, especially amines. This aspect has apparently not been studied at all. Liver cell synthesis and metabolism of many endogenous materials is also likely to be affected. Thus, the turnover of cholesterol, fatty acids, heme compounds, etc., which are certainly affected by phenobarbital, are likely to be changed by insecticides. We know that many of the effects of phenobarbital on hepatic steroid metabolism can be mimicked by chlorinated insecticides in both animals and man (see, for examples only (4,5); many other references could be cited).

The general area of chlorinated insecticide stimulation of drug metabolism is best known and needs the least comment. The principles can be reiterated, however: (1) animals or humans previously exposed to insecticides like DDT or chlordane may metabolize a variety of drugs and chemicals faster than before they were exposed to these insecticides. If the drug being used in such an insecticide-exposed person is inactivated by its metabolism by liver microsomes, then its action may be shorter and less intense. Indeed, the action may be so attenuated that therapeutic effect is lost. In a real sense, then, insecticide exposure may exacerbate a disease that was controlled by drugs before such exposure. Whether one can call this "environment" or more specifically, "insecticide-caused disease" is a semantic point, in my opinion; it is an adverse effect on health resulting from environment (insecticide) exposure.

If the drug being used in the insecticide-exposed person is activated by its metabolism by liver microsomes, then its effects may be made more intense and toxicity can occur at what used to be quite safe doses. Such results of enhanced toxicity are generally unexpected and

112

relatively hard to document in the literature. Drugs whose toxicity is likely to be enhanced by increasing their rate of metabolism are apparently rare (some cancer chemotherapeutic agents may belong here, as may some alkylated amines whose methyl or ethyl groups are removed during metabolism), but such effects of increased metabolism are not uncommon among a number of carcinogens and industrial solvents, especially those with an "affinity" for liver.

This latter phenomenon -- enhanced hepatotoxicity of chemicals after hepatic microsomal enzyme inhibition or induction -- has become increasingly important in studying the toxic potential for things like insecticides, air pollutants, etc., since many of these have been found to have stimulatory or inhibitory effects on these liver enzymes, or to change in toxicity when these enzymes are induced or inhibited by some other agent or chemical. Some of the first studies in this area were made using materials in rather less common use now than a few years ago.

The principle that appeared quickly, was that stimulation or inhibition of hepatic microsomal "drug-metabolizing" enzymes was associated with a marked change in the carcinogenicity or toxicity of chemicals like DMN (dimethylnitrosamine) or CCl_4 or $CHCl_3$ (6-9). Originally, the idea was that hepatic microsomal metabolism of things like CCl_4 could lead to toxic metabolites, and that stimulation of such metabolic pathways would lead to enhanced toxicity of these materials. Stimulation of microsomal enzymes by phenobarbital had effects (at least on $CHCl_3$ and CCl_4) similar to those of DDT, etc. (see for example ref. 8). A relatively non-toxic dose of something like CCl_4 became very hepatotoxic in animals pretreated with phenobarbital or DDT. This kind of interaction is a very active area of study in assessing "multiple factors in the causation of environmentally-induced disease," -- i.e., animals or man exposed to certain constituents of the environment may be much more susceptible to sub-toxic levels of other chemicals to which they are then exposed. The basis of this interaction can be via stimulation or inhibition of hepatic microsomal "drug-metabolizing" enzymes, depending on whether the parent toxic compound or its metabolite is more toxic. The chemical affecting the hepatic microsomal enzymes can be part of the environment. (DDT can be a stimulator of these enzymes; organophosphate insecticides and insecticide synergists such as piperonyl butoxide can be inhibitors of these enzymes (10, 11).) It may also be a drug (phenobarbital is an inducer and imipramine or SKF 525 are inhibitors). The agent causing the toxic effects may also be a part of the environment (organic solvents like CCl_4, or other insecticides or pesticides, or a fungal toxin like aflatoxin), or it may be a drug whose rate of metabolism is determining its action or toxicity. The combinations are obviously numerous, and the interactions may produce more or less of the effects of the toxic material(s).

The original clear understanding of how these interactions occur, and why the effects might change as doses, routes, animal species, and chemicals or agents are varied, has been muddied recently by the realization that alterations of hepatic microsomal enzymes may not be the only thing resulting from exposures to pesticides, pollutants or drugs; other things might also happen. I have already mentioned that inducers of hepatic microsomal "drug-metabolizing enzymes" cause changes in liver lipid (especially phospholipid) and protein contents. I have hinted at the fact that other liver functions such as excretion of bile or excretion of materials into bile, or blood flow through the liver might change (12,13). I have not mentioned that hepatic enzyme inducers may affect extrahepatic tissues like kidney, lung, or gut, and that all these things may happen at once, and with inhibitors of liver enzymes as well as stimulators. Absorption of materials from the gut can be altered by compounds like SKF 525A (14,15) which have been used as specific inhibitors of hepatic xenobiotic metabolism. The point is relatively familiar to the pharmacologist and toxicologist -- most chemicals affect several biological systems and usually in a dose-related manner. Which systems are affected and how much or how long will depend on whether the chemical gets there, in what quantity, and for how long. It is almost an axiom that any given effect of a chemical is usually of multiple causation, and to deal with this effect -- especially to alter it -- we must know which causes are most important. A given result may be caused by quite different actions; the similarity of what we see as these end results may impede our understanding of how to deal with their cause when these causes are different.

To conclude with some specific comments: phenobarbital, or organochlorine insecticides like DDT or chlordane, may change the action or toxicity of other chemicals including food additives, pollutants, other pesticides, and even drugs by changing the metabolism of these other chemicals by the liver. The same change in action may result from changing other aspects of disposition of these chemicals such as absorption, distribution (including storage), excretion, or interaction with receptor sitees. The environment may affect chemical and drug toxicity, chemicals and drugs may affect environmental toxicity, the environment may affect environmental toxicity. Thus, drugs can make pesticides more toxic or less toxic (16-18) and can affect body storage of pesticides (diphenylhydantoin reduces body residues of DDT (19). Pesticides can affect one another's toxicity and body storage (20,21), or toxicity or storage of other environmental constituents (e.g., piperonyl butoxide enhances storage of paraffins (22)), or of drugs (already referenced several times). The mechanisms for many of these interactions are believed to be understood and seem to involve changing hepatic microsomal xenobiotic metabolizing systems. I would close by saying that this may or may not be true, but it offers a starting point for much further study and concern.

REFERENCES

1. Fouts, J. R. (1970). Some effects of insecticides on hepatic microsomal enzymes in various animal species. Rev. Canad. Biol. 29: 377.

2. Fouts, J. R. (1970). The stimulation and inhibition of hepatic microsomal drug metabolizing enzymes with special reference to effects of environmental contaminants. Toxicol. Appl. Pharmacol. 17: 804.

3. Schaffner, F. and Popper, H. (1969). Cholestasis is the result of hypoactive hypertrophic smooth endoplasmic reticulum in the hepatocyte. Lancet 1: 355.

4. Kupfer, D. (1969). Influence of chlorinated hydrocarbons and organophosphate insecticides on metabolism of steroids. Ann. N. Y. Acad. Sci. 160: 244.

5. Poland, A. et al. (1970). Effect of intensive occupational exposure to DDT on phenylbutazone and cortisol metabolism in human subjects. Clin. Pharmacol. Therap. 11: 724.

6. McLean, A. E. M. and Vorschuuren, H. G. (1969). Effects of diet and microsomal enzyme induction on the toxicity of dimethyl nitrosamine. Brit. J. Exptl. Pathol. 50: 22.

7. McLean, E. K., McLean, A. E. M. and Sutton, P. M. (1969). Instant cirrhosis. An improved method for producing cirrhosis of the liver in rats by simultaneous administration of carbon tetrachloride and phenobarbitone. Brit. J. Exptl. Pathol. 50: 502.

8. McLean, A. E. M. (1970). The effect of protein deficiency and microsomal enzyme induction by DDT and phenobarbitone on the acute toxicity of chloroform and a pyrrolizidine alkaloid, retrorsine. Brit. J. Exptl. Pathol. 51: 317.

9. Brodie, B. B. et al. (1971). Possible mechanism of liver necrosis caused by aromatic organic compounds. Proc. Natl. Acad. Sci. 68: 160.

10. Fujii, K. et al. (1970). Structure-activity relations for methylene-dioxyphenyl and related compounds on hepatic microsomal enzyme function, as measured by prolongation of hexobarbital

narcosis and zoxazolamine paralysis in mice. Toxicol. Appl. Pharmacol. 16: 482.

11. Hart, L. G. and Fouts, J. R. (1963). Effects of acute and chronic DDT administration on hepatic microsomal drug metabolism in the rat. Proc. Soc. Exptl. Biol. Med. 114: 388.

12. Klaassen, C. D. and Plaa, G. L. (1968). Studies on the mechanism of phenobarbital-enhanced sulfobromphthalein disappearance. J. Pharmacol. Exptl. Therap. 161: 361.

13. Levine, W. G. et al. (1970). The role of the hepatic endoplasmic reticulum in the biliary excretion of foreign compounds by the rat. Biochem. Pharmacol. 19: 235.

14. Marchand, C., McLean, S. and Plaa, G. L. (1970). The effect of SKF 525A on the distribution of carbon tetrachloride in rats. J. Pharmacol. Exptl. Therap. 174: 232.

15. McLean, S. and Marchand, C. (1970). The effect of SKF 525A on drug concentration in the blood. Life Sci. 9: 1075.

16. DuBois, K. P. and Kinoshita, F. K. (1968). Influence of induction of hepatic microsomal enzymes by phenobarbital on toxicity of organic phosphate insecticides. Proc. Soc. Exptl. Biol. Med. 129: 699.

17. Menzer, R. E. and Best, N. H. (1968). Effect of phenobarbital on the toxicity of several organophosphorous insecticides. Toxicol. Appl. Pharmacol. 13: 37.

18. Selye, H. (1970). Resistance to various pesticides induced by catatoxic steroids. Arch. Env. Health 21: 706.

19. Davies, J. E. et al. (1969). Effect of anticonvulsant drugs on dicophane (DDT) residues in man. Lancet 1: 7.

20. Menzer, R. E. (1970). Effect of chlorinated hydrocarbons in the diet on the toxicity of several organophosphorous insecticides. Toxicol. Appl. Pharmacol. 16: 446.

21. Street, J. C. and Blau, A. D. (1966). Insecticide interactions affecting residue accumulation in animal tissues. Toxicol. Appl. Pharmacol. 8: 497.

22. Albro, P. W. and Fishbein, L. (1970). Short-term effects of piperonyl butoxide on the disposition of dietary hydrocarbon in rat tissues. Life Sci. 9: 729.

CHAPTER 9. DRUG-CHEMICAL INTERACTIONS AS A FACTOR IN ENVIRONMENTALLY INDUCED DISEASE

JERRY R. MITCHELL and JAMES R. GILLETTE,
National Heart and Lung Institute, Bethesda, Maryland

"Environmentally induced disease" is not an isolated problem. It must be considered in context with the exposure of man and animals to all foreign compounds, whether these are present normally in the environment, adventitious contaminants in food, inhaled from the atmosphere, or administered therapeutically. We are confronted with a profusion of chemicals in the form of industrial and municipal wastes, air and water pollutants, herbicides, pesticides, cosmetics, food additives, and drugs administered over extended periods of time. Yet, because of the lack of a biochemical-physiological framework on which to base cause and effect mechanisms, we often do not know what these substances do to biological systems. Nevertheless, the fundamental questions remain the same: (1) How is the foreign substance absorbed into and eliminated from the body? (2) Does the foreign substance cause deleterious effects and, if so, how?

In evaluating these questions, it should be realized that a substance may appear to be innocuous when encountered alone, but toxic after repeated exposures or in combination with other substances. This aspect of the problem of "multiple factors in the causation of environmentally induced diseases" is the topic we wish to discuss.

Interactions of chemicals and drugs to produce adverse effects may be divided arbitrarily into five categories: (1) Direct drug-chemical interactions (alteration of a drug's access to or activity at its site of action by another compound); (2) Sensitization by repeated exposure; (3) Alteration of renal excretion; (4) Alteration of hepatic metabolism; and (5) Induction of metabolism as a cause of structural and biochemical tissue damage.

DIRECT DRUG-CHEMICAL INTERACTIONS

A dramatic example of the complex interrelationships between therapeutic agents and foreign substances is the severe and occasionally lethal hypertensive crisis or cardiac arrhythmia that occurs when individuals who are treated with monoamine oxidase inhibitors eat certain cheeses, beers, wines, or herring containing large quantities of tyramine (1). The same interaction occurs with other sympathomimetic amines present in over-the-counter nasal decongestants or cold remedies, and especially with amphetamine appetite-suppressants and "pep pills" (2,3). To further complicate matters, a patient may receive a monoamine oxidase inhibitor unwittingly. Thus, furazolidone, an antibacterial agent used in the treatment of various bacterial and protozoal infections, recently was shown to be converted in vivo in man to a compound that is a potent inhibitor of monoamine oxidase (4).

Certain drugs may induce disease by preventing the absorption of environmental nutrients and vitamins. The occurrence of megaloblastic anemia in patients receiving diphenylhydantoin (5), in other patients who are receiving oral contraceptive agents (6), and in some patients with chronic alcoholism (7), is due to a deficiency of folic acid in these people. The mechanisms of this anemia are traceable to the fact that the first two drugs inhibit the deconjugation of the poorly absorbed polyglutamate form of folic acid to the readily absorbed monoglutamate, while alcohol appears to produce a mucosal blockade of folic acid absorption. Malabsorption of vitamin B_{12}, carotene and various fats also has been reported after administration of neomycin, colchicine, and para-aminosalicylic acid (8). In addition, drugs themselves often are poorly absorbed because of drug-chemical interactions. Antacids sold over-the-counter are commonly considered harmless and frequently are taken in conjunction with drugs. Both aluminum hydroxide and magnesium hydroxide decrease the absorption of tetracyclines, pentobarbital, and many acidic drugs such as phenylbutazone (9).

Other examples of direct drug-chemical interactions include antihypertensive agents, such as guanethidine and bethanidine, which must be accumulated into adrenergic neurons by an active transport system in order to exert their pharmacologic effect. Desipramine and protriptyline, tricyclic antidepressants, inhibit the uptake of guanethidine and bethanidine by the neuron and thus prevent their antihypertensive action, a potentially disastrous drug-drug interaction (10).

SENSITIZATION BY REPEATED EXPOSURE

Approximately 2% of the population receiving penicillin develop allergic reactions; these account for 10% of all allergic drug reactions. Annually, some 200 of these reactions are anaphylactoid, resulting in over 60 deaths. Clearly, penicillin's ubiquitous presence is responsible for the high incidence of sensitization. Dairy products frequently contain an appreciable amount of penicillin. Fish, fowl, and pork are preserved with various antibiotics, including penicillin. Antimicrobial agents fed to cattle and other animals for medicinal purposes may induce sensitization when the meat of the animal is ingested. Furthermore, sensitization to penicillin often sensitizes to the cephalosporin group of antibiotics as well.

Then there is a multitude of nitrogenous aromatic compounds which are potent sensitizers. This group consists of aniline and derivatives, naphthylamines, diamines, sulfonamides, sulfones, aminobenzoic acid and derivatives, aminosalicylic acid, various nitro-compounds and aminoazo dyes. The large number of compounds represented here has many diversified uses in our lives. They serve as important starting materials or intermediates for the synthesis of numerous chemical substances, especially medicines and dyes. Aniline, toluidine, and other liquid aromatic amines are used as solvents in technical processes as well as in finished products. Most photographic developers contain aromatic amines

and aminophenols. Diamines, particularly
p-phenylenediamine and its derivatives, serve as
oxidative dyes for hair and furs. The majority of
synthetic dyes are manufactured from aromatic amines;
many of the finished and most commonly used azo dyes
contain nitro groups or free and substituted amino
groups. Technically used dyes often retain
appreciable amounts of aromatic amines as impurities.
In the past, aminoazo dyes have been used in the
coloring of cosmetics, drugs, clothing, and foods
such as butter, beverages, candies, and fruits. The
FDA has removed most of those which were absorbed and
metabolized, although a few such as tartrazine
persist.

The allergic manifestations produced by aromatic
nitrogenous compounds are, in most instances,
restricted to the contact type of sensitization (11).
However, some of them can sensitize certain
mesenchymal systems and thereby produce atopic
allergies, such as rhinitis, asthma, urticaria, or
intestinal disturbances. A few, especially
p-phenylenediamine and certain sulfonamides, are able
to sensitize almost any cell system.

Worst of all, allergic sensitization to one
compound frequently extends to numerous other ones
within the group. Thus, a patient sensitized by the
p-phenylenediamine dye on her fur coat may show
severe reactions on administration of a
sulfonamide, or of a local anesthetic such as
benzocaine (aminobenzoic acid derivative), or when
she encounters certain azo-dyes or aniline
derivatives. Indeed, Meltzer and Baer (12) have
reported one patient with atopic dermatitis to
benzocaine, who subsequently developed a vesicular
eruption after treatment with a sulfonamide, and
again a few years later after use of a commercial
sunburn preventive containing the monoglycerol ester
of p-aminobenzoic acid. A series of skin tests
revealed that the patient was allergic to virtually
every substance in the group of aromatic nitrogenous
compounds! Similarly, a constant worry when
treating tuberculous patients concomitantly with
para-aminosalicylic acid and isoniazid is the
possibility that sensitization to para-aminosalicylic
acid, which occurs in about 7% of the patients,
occasionally may extend to isoniazid, the keystone
in the chemotherapy of tuberculosis (13).

122

ALTERATION OF RENAL EXCRETION

The excretion rates of many drugs are altered by changing the pH of urine. These alterations assume clinical significance when the renal excretion of free drug is a major pathway for elimination of the drug. In man, weak acids such as aspirin, salicylate, and phenobarbital, are excreted more rapidly in alkaline urine, while weak bases, such as quinidine and amphetamine, are excreted more quickly in acid urine (14,15,16). It is obvious that an inadequate response to standard doses of these drugs, or problems of toxicity from overdosage (especially with quinidine), will result whenever the diet of these patients includes sufficient amounts of sodium bicarbonate, acid ash, or cranberry juice. Perhaps the greatest threat comes from a new health fad -- self-pollution with large quantities of vitamin C, a potent urinary acidifying agent!

Some drugs also are eliminated from the body by active renal tubular secretion. Concurrent administration of another drug similarly secreted may delay elimination with resulting accumulation and toxicity. For example, salicylate and other anions can slow the rate of methotrexate excretion (17). Likewise, hypoglycemia after acetohexamide is potentiated by the concomitant administration of phenylbutazone, which interferes with the tubular secretion of an active hypoglycemic metabolite of acetohexamide (18). Therapeutic advantage of this type of interaction is taken when probenecid is given with penicillin to prolong effective plasma concentrations of the latter.

ALTERATION OF HEPATIC METABOLISM

INHIBITION -- Drug-metabolizing microsomal enzymes of a variety of animal species are inhibited by many compounds. In recent years, it has been recognized that one drug can also inhibit the metabolism of another in man and thereby increase the magnitude of the pharmacologic effect. For example, phenylbutazone (19) and sulfaphenazole (20) reduce the rate of metabolism of tolbutamide and thus potentiate the hypoglycemic response. Similarly, the metabolism of diphenylhydantoin is decreased by isoniazid (21), bishydroxycoumarin (22a), and methylphenidate (23). Concurrent therapy with diphenylhydantoin and any of these agents may produce serious diphenylhydantoin toxicity with permanent cerebellar dysfunction. Phenyramidol inhibits the metabolism of bishydroxycoumarin, diphenylhydantoin, and tolbutamide (22a,b,24). Severe hemorrhage has occurred when patients anticoagulated with bishydroxycoumarin were treated with phenyramidol.

INDUCTION -- Several hundred compounds are known to induce the synthesis of microsomal drug-metabolizing enzymes in animals and in man. Indeed, this has been one of the most active areas of research on "multiple factors in the causation of environmentally induced disease." Since other participants will discuss much of this work, no further elaboration is necessary here. In addition, several thorough reviews of this subject are available (25-29).

However, it should be pointed out that induction of metabolism by drugs is not necessarily adverse in itself, and can have therapeutic application. Treatment with phenobarbital is successful in reducing the unconjugated hyperbilirubinemia of some patients with an associated deficiency of bilirubin glucuronyl transferase activity (30). Diphenylhydantoin stimulates the microsomal hydroxylation of cortisol and has been used in man to treat Cushing's syndrome (31). Induction of metabolism by DDT or drugs like phenobarbital can prevent the acute toxicity and carcinogenicity of aflatoxin B_1 and perhaps other aflatoxins (32).

INDUCTION OF METABOLISM AS A CAUSE OF TISSUE DAMAGE

While much has been written about the ability of many drugs and environmental chemicals to induce their own as well as other compounds' metabolism, drug metabolism as a cause of drug toxicity has been largely ignored. Although drugs and environmental toxins generally are converted in the body to derivatives that are less toxic than the parent substances, many chemically inert organic compounds are transformed in vivo to potent alkylating agents which combine with tissue proteins and nucleic acids to produce allergies, tissue lesions, genetic mutations, or cancer (33-36). Since exposure to enzyme inducers like phenobarbital and DDT can dramatically convert many of these substances from nontoxic to lethal compounds, it is obviously important to expand our investigations of these interactions and to explore the possibility that tissue damage produced by therapeutic agents is mediated by reactive metabolites as well.

What little is known about metabolism as a cause of toxicity stems primarily from studies on biochemical mechanisms of liver injury. Since the activity of hepatic microsomal enzymes in producing toxic metabolites is related to nutritional control, as well as to the effects of enzyme inducers and inhibitors, studies determining the effects on hepatotoxicity of treatments which alter the metabolism of known hepatotoxins have been particularly fruitful. Thus, the feeding of a low protein diet almost abolishes the lethal and hepatotoxic effects of carbon tetrachloride. This effect is reversed by administration of DDT or phenobarbital (32). Similarly, enzyme induction by DDT and phenobarbital render rats more sensitive to the lethal and hepatotoxic actions of chloroform.

Recent studies in our laboratory indicate that the centrolobular liver necrosis produced in rats by bromobenzene, and a number of other halogenated aromatic hydrocarbons, also is mediated through a chemically reactive metabolite: phenobarbital pretreatment stimulates the metabolism of bromobenzene and markedly potentiates the liver necrosis, while SKF 525A blocks the metabolism of bromobenzene and prevents the liver necrosis (34,37,38). Biochemical evidence suggests that the active intermediate of bromobenzene is an epoxide, which initially reacts with glutathione in hepatocytes to yield glutathione-bromobenzene conjugates, thereby depleting hepatocytes of glutathione. Since a function of glutathione is to protect nucleophilic sites in tissues from electrophilic attack (39), it is likely that the continued formation of epoxide in the absence of glutathione • favors alkylation of tissue macromolecules, producing tissue damage. In accord with this view, administration of cysteine, the

125

precursor of glutathione, protects rats against bromobenzene-induced hepatic necrosis (40), while necrosis is markedly enhanced by prior administration of diethyl maleate (37) and other substances which deplete the liver of glutathione. (The latter interactions, of course, illustrate the type of direct drug-chemical interactions outlined above.)

Another carefully studied hepatotoxin is dimethylnitrosamine, which requires demethylation by microsomal enzymes before it exerts its toxic and carcinogenic effects. In protein-depleted animals, dimethylnitrosamine's metabolism is greatly reduced in the liver but unaffected in the kidney. The decreased liver clearance of dimethylnitrosamine allows more dimethylnitrosamine to come into contact with the kidneys. This changes the action specturm of dimethylnitrosamine; instead of a lethal hepatotoxic effect, the protein-deficient rats escape immediate death from severe liver necrosis only to die twelve months later from kidney tumors (32).

Because of these studies with dimethylnitrosamine, we recently have turned our attention to acetaminophen, a drug which produces acute centrolobular hepatic necrosis and renal tubular necrosis in man (41) and in rats (42) when taken in huge doses. This analgesic now rivals aspirin in sales over-the-counter in many European countries and in Australia. As the major metabolite of phenacetin, it also has been implicated in the "analgesic nephropathy syndrome" prevalent in these countries.

We have found in rats that induction of the metabolism of acetaminophen by phenobarbital and 3-methylcholanthrene markedly potentiates hepatic necrosis (Mitchell, Brodie and Gillette, unpublished). That these data may be directly applicable to man is suggested by the finding of an increased susceptibility to acetaminophen-induced hepatic necrosis in patients using barbiturates or ethanol (41). Since the microsomal enzymes in the kidney are similar to those in the liver, the possibility that analgesic nephropathy may result from a toxic metabolite generated in the kidney is obvious. If this is so, the geographic occurrence of the disease may be related to the diet of the residents, to their exposure to insecticide inducers, to their use of ethanol, or to the practice of combining inducers such as caffeine and antipyrine in the analgesic mixtures.

SUMMARY

A variety of foods and environmental chemicals interact with therapeutic agents to produce adverse effects. These interactions have been discussed as a factor in environmentally induced disease. Interactions between drugs also are discussed when the use of the drugs in our society is sufficiently widespread to consider the drugs as part of the environment (e.g., antacids, ethanol, penicillin, salicylates, vitamin C). No attempt is made to include those drug-drug interactions of concern primarily to physicians, except as an occasional illustration of a particular type of novel interaction. Special emphasis is given to drug metabolism as a cause of biochemical and structural tissue damage, because we believe that the implications of drug-chemical interactions in this area have not been adequately considered by the health sciences community.

REFERENCES

1. Sjöqvist, F. (1965). Psychotropic drugs. 2. Interaction between monoamine oxidase (MAO) inhibitors and other substances, Proc. Roy. Soc. Med. 58: 967.

2. Cuthbert, M. F., Greenberg, M. P. and Morley, S. W. (1969). Cough and cold remedies: A potential danger to patients on monoamine oxidase inhibitors. Brit. Med. J. 1: 404.

3. Pettinger, W. A. and Oates, J. A. (1968). Supersensitivity to tyramine during monoamine oxidase inhibition in man. Clin. Pharmacol. Therap. 9: 341.

4. Pettinger, W. A., Soyangco, F. C. and Oates, J. A. (1968). Inhibition of monoamine oxidase in man by furazolidone. Clin. Pharmacol. Therap. 9: 442.

5. Reynolds, E. H. et al. (1965). Reversible absorptive defects in anticonvulsant megaloblastic anemia. J. Clin. Pathol. 18: 593.

6. Streiff, R. R. (1970). Folate deficiency and oral contraceptives. J. Amer. Med. Assoc. 214: 105.

7. Halsted, C. H., Griggs, R. C. and Harris, J. W. (1967). The effect of alcoholism on the absorption of folic acid (^{3}H-PGA) evaluated by plasma levels and urine excretion. J. Lab. Clin. Med. 69: 116.

8. Faloon, W. W. (1970). Drug production of intestinal malabsorption. N. Y. State J. Med. 70: 2189.

9. Swidler, G. (1971). Handbook of Drug Interactions. Wiley-Interscience, New York, 21.

10. Mitchell, J. R. et al. (1970). Guanethidine and related agents. III. Antagonism by drugs which inhibit the norepinephrine pump in man. J. Clin. Invest. 49: 1596.

11. Fisher, A. A. (1967). Contact Dermatitis. Lea and Febiger, Philadelphia.

12. Meltzer, L. and Baer, R. L. (1949). Sensitization to monoglycerol para-aminobenzoate. J. Invest. Dermatol. 12: 31.

13. Klatskin, G. (1968). In: L. Schiff, (ed.), Diseases of the Liver. Lippincott, Philadelphia, 543.

14. Hollister, L. and Levy, G. (1965). Some aspects of salicylate distribution and metabolism in man. J. Pharmacol. Sci. 54: 1126.

15. Gerhardt, R. E. et al. (1969). Quinidine excretion in aciduria and alkaluria. Ann. Int. Med. 71: 927.

16. Davis, J. M. et al. (1971). Effects of urinary pH on amphetamine metabolism, Ann. N. Y. Acad. Sci. 179: 493.

17. Liegler, D. G. et al. (1969). The effect of organic acids on renal clearance of methotrexate in man. Clin. Pharmacol. Therap. 10: 849.

18. Field, J. B. et al. (1967). Potentiation of acetohexamide hypoglycemia by phenylbutazone. New Eng. J. Med. 277: 889.

19. Gulbrandsen, R. (1959). Potentiation of tolbutamide by phenylbutazone. Tiddskr. Norske Laegefo. 79: 1127.

20. Christensen, L. K., Hansen, J. M. and Kristensen, M. (1963). Sulphaphenazole-induced hypoglycaemic attacks in tolbutamide-treated diabetics. Lancet 2: 1298.

21. Kutt, H., Winters, W. and McDowell, F. H. (1966). Depression of parahydroxylation of diphenylhydantoin by antituberculosis chemotherapy. Neurology 16: 594.

22a. Solomon, H. M. and Schrogie, J. J. (1967). The effect of phenyramidol on the metabolism of diphenylhydantoin. Clin. Pharmacol. Therap. 8: 554.

22b. Solomon, H. M. and Schrogie, J. J. (1967). Effect of phenyramidol and bishydroxycoumarin on the metabolism of tolbutamide in human subjects. Metabolism 16: 1029.

23. Garrettson, L, K., Perel, J. M. and Dayton, P. G. (1969). Methylphenidate interaction with both anticonvulsants and ethyl biscoumacetate. J. Amer. Med. Assoc. 207: 2053.

24. Solomon, H. M. and Schrogie, J. J. (1966). The effect of phenyramidol on the metabolism of bishydroxycoumarin. J. Pharmacol. Exptl. Therap. 154: 660.

25. Gillette, J. R. (1963). Metabolism of drugs and other foreign compounds by enzymatic mechanisms. Progr. Drug Res. 6: 11.

26. Conney, A. H. (1967). Pharmacological implications of microsomal enzyme induction. Pharmacol. Rev. 19: 317.

27. Kuntzman, R. (1969). Drugs and enzyme induction. Ann. Rev. Pharmacol. 9: 21.

28. Fouts, J. R. (1970). Some effects of insecticides on hepatic microsomal enzymes in various animal species. Rev. Can. Biol. 29: 377.

29. Conney, A. H. et al. (1971). Effects of environmental chemicals on the metabolism of drugs, carcinogens, and normal body constituents in man. Ann. N. Y. Acad. Sci. 179: 155.

30. Arias, I. M. et al. (1969). Chronic non-hemolytic unconjugated hyperbilirubinemia with glucuronyl transferase deficiency. Amer. J. Med. 47: 395.

31. Werk, E. E., Sholiton, L. J. and Olinger, C. P. (1966). Amelioration of non-tumorous Cushing's syndrome by diphenylhydantoin. 2nd Int. Congr. Hormonal Steroids, Milan Abstracts Int. Congr. Ser. No. III. Excerpta Medical Foundation, New York, 301.

32. Judah, J. D., McLean, A. E. M. and McLean, E. K. (1970). Biochemical mechanisms of liver injury. Amer. J. Med. 49: 609.

33. Levine, B. B. (1966). Immunochemical mechanisms of drug allergy. Ann. Rev. Med. 17: 23.

34. Brodie, B. B. et al. (1971). Possible mechanism of liver necrosis caused by aromatic organic compounds. Proc. Nat. Acad. Sci. 68: 160.

35. Ames, B. N. (1971). The detection of chemical mutagens with enteric bacteria. In: A. Hollaender, (ed.), Chemical Mutagens: Principles and Methods for their Detection. Plenum, New York, 267.

36. Miller, E. C. and Miller, J. A. (1966). Mechanisms of chemical carcinogenesis: Nature of proximate carcinogens and interactions with macromolecules. Pharmacol. Rev. 18: 805.

37. Reid, W. D. et al. (1971). Bromobenzene metabolism and hepatic necrosis. Pharmacol. 6: 41.

38. Mitchell, J. R. et al. (1971). Bromobenzene-induced hepatic necrosis: Species differences and protection by SKF 525A. Res. Com. Chem. Pathol. Pharmacol. 2: 877.

39. Boyland, E. and Chasseaud, L. F. (1969). The role of glutathione and glutathione S-transferases in mercapturic acid biosynthesis. Adv. Enzymol. 32: 173.

40. Koch-Weser, D. et al. (1953). Hepatic necrosis due to bromobenzene as an example of conditioned amino acid deficiency. Metabolism 2: 248.

41. Prescott, L. F. et al. (1971). Plasma-paracetamol half-life and hepatic necrosis in patients with paracetamol over-dosage. Lancet 1: 519.

42. Boyd, E. M. and Bereczky, G. M. (1966). Liver necrosis from paracetamol. Brit. J. Pharmacol. 26: 606.

PART III

COMPLICATIONS INTRODUCED BY
STORAGE OF CAUSATIVE AGENTS

Storage and release in themselves constitute a complex system, with numerous stages and opportunities for perturbation, as indicated in the following very much simplified diagram.

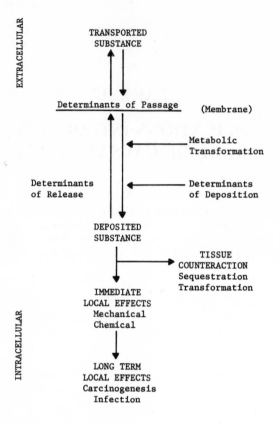

EXTRACELLULAR

TRANSPORTED
SUBSTANCE

Determinants of Passage   (Membrane)

Metabolic
Transformation

Determinants   Determinants
of Release   of Deposition

DEPOSITED
SUBSTANCE

TISSUE
COUNTERACTION
Sequestration
Transformation

IMMEDIATE
LOCAL EFFECTS
Mechanical
Chemical

INTRACELLULAR

LONG TERM
LOCAL EFFECTS
Carcinogenesis
Infection

This is clearly a dynamic system and one would need
to know the kinetics at each stage for thorough
understanding.

Contributors were asked to discuss certain
well-known instances where a causative agent may be
stored in body tissues and subsequently released into
the general circulation. From what they have to say
it is clear that we are still a long way from having
the quantitative data that would permit a predictive
measure of probable events.

CHAPTER 10. ROLE OF BODY STORES IN ENVIRONMENTALLY INDUCED DISEASE – DDT AND LEAD

WAYLAND J. HAYES, JR., ROBERT A. NEAL, and HAROLD H. SANDSTEAD, Vanderbilt University School of Medicine, Nashville, Tennessee

It has been known for many years that several toxic elements are found regularly in food, water, and human tissue. Such toxic elements not known to be beneficial at any dosage include lead, mercury, and arsenic. Some other toxic elements are found only at barely detectable concentrations or only in people with occupational or other special exposure. Of the toxic environmental elements, lead probably has received the greatest attention over a period of years.

The occurrences in human tissue of various organic compounds derived from food, drugs, or tobacco has been recognized for many years also. However, DDT apparently was the first synthetic organic compound demonstrated in the tissues of people who did not acquire it through occupational exposure or as a drug. It is of interest that, as a result of search using improved techniques, equally old compounds such as hexachlorophene, or certain older compounds such as the polychlorinated biphenyls and pentachlorophenol, have now been demonstrated in people with only environmental exposure. No doubt further search would reveal other old compounds. Search has already revealed the storage of many new materials, notably the chlorinated hydrocarbon insecticides introduced after DDT. However, the storage of DDT in man has been the subject of more extensive study than that of any other synthetic organic compound encountered in the environment.

It is reasonable to choose DDT as a synthetic compound widely dispersed in the environment and to choose lead as a toxic element also widely dispersed.

DDT

STORAGE OF DDT IN MAN

DDT in Adipose Tissue

From the mid-1950s onward there has been an apparent decrease in the storage of DDT in the fat of people in the general population of the United States of America (See Fig. 1). Some caution must be exercised in interpreting the results because the early sets of samples were small and the method of chemical analysis changed about 1962. Perhaps even more important, the samples were taken without any plan regarding geographical distribution. It became apparent only gradually that the values obtained tended to increase from north to south. However, it was shown: (a) that an astonishingly accurate estimate of DDT storage in human population was obtained by examining a small subset (90); and (b) that analyses by the Schechter-Haller and gas chromatographic methods of pairs of aliquots from the same extracts give satisfactory agreement (1-3). The observed decrease in the concentration of DDT in food (4-6) offers an adequate reason for the decrease in storage in people. Finally, the apparent rate of decrease from an average level of about 6 ppm of p,p'-DDT and about 16 ppm of total DDT-related compounds in 1955 was considerably slower than the rate of decrease from about 300 ppm observed experimentally in man (7). The slower rate of decrease at a lower rate of storage is exactly what would be predicted on the basis of animal experiments. Therefore, there is reason to believe that the observed decrease in storage of DDT in the general population of the United States of America is real.

Storage of DDT has now been measured in the fat of people living not only in North America [Canada (20,21) and U. S. A. (1,8-19,22,23)], but also South America [Venezuela (24)]; Europe [Belgium (25), Czechoslovakia (26), Denmark (27), England (18,28-32), France (33), Germany (34,35), Hungary (36), Italy (37), Netherlands (38,39), Poland (40),

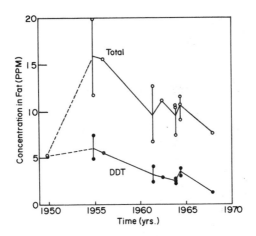

Fig. 1. Concentration of DDT (solid points) and of all DDT-related materials (open circles) in the body fat of people in the general population. The curve is drawn through the mean of means for surveys made in the same year. As indicated by the dotted lines, it is not certain whether the value measured in 1950 represents DDT or total DDT-related material. The values shown are from unpublished reports of the U. S. Public Health Service as well as from published reports from various sources (1, 7-19).

Roumania (41), Spain (42)]; Asia [India (2), Israel (43,44)]; Africa [Nigeria (45)]; and Oceania [Australia (46,47) and New Zealand (48)]. The highest values were found among the civilian population of India, the average for p,p'-DDT and total DDT-related material being 16 and 39 ppm, respectively (2).

DDT has been found in all human populations when it was sought. There is some tendency for the storage levels to be higher in warm countries where insects present a greater problem in agriculture. A similar trend may be observed in connection with the warmer and cooler parts of the United States of America. Whether the difference reflects the degree of household use of pesticides, or the use of locally raised food, or even a physiological difference in absorption is not known. Furthermore, not all differences in storage are secondary to temperature. Levels of DDT in human adipose tissue or milk from Russia and countries under Russian influence are relatively high. There is considerable reason to think that differences between the storage observed in civilian and military populations in India were associated with direct application of DDT to stored food.

Although it may not be possible to explain the exact degree of storage of DDT observed in each country, there is nothing in the observed facts to suggest that the differences do not correspond with differences in exposure. This basic conclusion is reinforced by a study of storage in people with occupational, special environmental, or other special exposure to the insecticide as summarized in Table 1. Meat abstainers (11) and Eskimos (49), whose diets are relatively free of DDT, store significantly less of it than most people do. On the other hand, people with occupational exposure to the compound store more (11,50,51). Apparently the highest recorded storage of DDT-related materials in a healthy man was 648 ppm of DDT plus 434 ppm of DDE measured in the fat of a formulator (10). However, the total value was not much more than that involving 657 ppm of DDT and 156 ppm of DDE measured in a man who had received p,p'-DDT at a rate of 35 mg/day for 21.5 months (7).

DDT in Other Tissues and Fluids

It is expected that an absorbed compound will be distributed to all tissues, although often in very different concentrations. As reviewed elsewhere (53), it was shown by early experiments in animals that DDT in fact does reach all organs and that it or its metabolites may be found in all excreta. A complete demonstration of this distribution in people of the general population had to await the development of more sensitive analytical methods because the concentrations of DDT in nonadipose tissues and in excreta are low unless dosage is high. However, the distribution of DDT in various nonadipose tissues of people with ordinary exposure has been measured for several years, the earliest reports being as follows: blood, 1966 (32,54); various organs, 1965 (55); and the fetus, 1962 (36).

Although DDA was found many years ago in the urine of a volunteer (56) and in the urine of some people in the general population (57), it was not possible until recently to detect it in the urine of

TABLE 1 -- CONCENTRATION OF DDT-DERIVED MATERIAL IN BODY FAT OF PEOPLE IN THE UNITED STATES WITH SPECIAL EXPOSURE (ENVIRONMENTAL, OCCUPATIONAL, OR DIETARY) to DDT[a]

Exposure	Year	No. of Samples	DDT (ppm)	DDE as DDT (ppm)	Total as DDT (ppm)	DDE as DDT (% of total)	Reference
Died before DDT	<1942	10	b	b	b	-	(11)
Environmental[c]	1954-1956	110	6.0	9.6	15.6	62	(11)
Environmental[c]	1961-1962	28	4.3	8.6	12.9	67	(16)
Applicators	1954-1956	30	14.0	21.1	35.1	60	(16)
Applicators	1961-1962	14	10.7	24.1	34.8	69	(16)
Formulator	1951	1	122	141	263	54	(52)
Formulator	1954	1	648	483	1131	43	(10)
Meat abstainers	1955-1956	16	2.3	3.6	5.9	61	(11)
Eskimos[d]	1960	20	0.8	2.2	3.0	73	(49)
Volunteers given 3.5 mg per day orally[e]	1953-1954	2	30	3.9	34	11	(10)
Volunteers given 3.5 mg per day orally[f]	1957-1958	6	50	21	71	30	(7)
Volunteers given 35 mg per day orally[e]	1953-1954	6	234	24	258	9	(10)
Volunteers given 35 mg per day orally[f]	1957-1958	6	281	40	321	12	(7)

a Colorimetric.
b Not detected.
c Residents of the Wenatchee, Wash. area living within 500 ft. of agricultural application.
d Alaskan eskimos who ate predominately a native diet shown to contain little or no DDT.
e Based on samples taken after 11 months or more of dosage.
f Based on samples taken after 21.5 months of dosage.

TABLE 2 -- CONCENTRATION OF DDT-DERIVED MATERIAL IN HUMAN MILK

Country	Year	No. of Samples	Analytical Method	DDT (ppm)	DDE as DDT (ppm)	Total as DDT	DDE as DDT (% of total)	Reference
United States	1950	32	Color	0.13	-	0.13	-	(15)
United States	1960-1961	10	Color	0.08	0.04	0.12[b]	33	(60)
United States	1962	6	Color	0-0.2[a]	0.025[a]	<0.37[b]	-	(61)
United States	1968		GLC	0.026	0.047	0.078	60	(62)
Hungary	1963	10	Color	0.13-0.26[a]	-	-	-	(63)
England	1963-1964	19[c]	GLC	0.05	0.08	0.13	62	(30)
Russia	1964	16	Color	1.22-4.88	-	-	-	(64)
Italy	1965?	2[d]	GLC	0.001	0.05	0.055	-	(37)
Poland	1966	26	Color	0.27	-	-	62	(65)
Poland	1967	25	Color	0.40	-	-	58	(65)
Sweden	1967?	-	-	-	-	0.117	-	(66)
Russia	1968?	4505	-	0.1-1.0	-	-	-	(67)
Belgium	1968?	20	GLC	0.05	-	-	-	(68)
Czechoslovakia	1968			0.101	-	-	-	(69)
Russia	1969?	370	TLC	0.1	-	-	-	(70)

a Range of values for milk containing 4% fat containing 3.3 to 6.6 ppm.
b Maximal value.
c These samples also contained 0.013 ppm BHC and 0.006 ppm dieldrin.
d Samples reported to contain 0.001 ppm aldrin, as unlikely finding.

all persons in the general population. In 1967 it
became possible to demonstrate DDT and several of its
metabolites, notably DDE, in the urine of essentially
every person (58). Still later, a method was
developed to measure DDA at the low concentrations
found in many samples; the mean is found to be 0.014
ppm, that is just below the sensitivity of the old
method (59).

The occurrence of DDT in human milk was reported
in connection with the first survey of DDT in the
general population (15). Since then, the occurrence
of DDT in human milk has been noted in several
countries (See Table 2). In 1965 it was reported
from both England (30) and the United States of
America (60) that the concentration of DDT in human
milk is greater than that in cow's milk. That is,
of course, exactly what one would expect as between
an omnivor and a herbivor. In any event, the
authors gave the fact little emphasis, although
Quinby and his colleagues (60) did point out that a
lactating woman apparently is in negative DDT
balance. Recently certain authors have given an
unreasonable emphasis to the difference in the
concentrations in human milk and cow's milk,
rather than emphasizing that the concentration in
both kinds of milk is low in most countries. The
exception is that high concentrations have been
reported in the milk of Russian and, to a lesser
degree, Polish women. The concentrations in Russia
appear to have decreased recently, but in the USA
they have remained essentially stable.

EFFECT OF DDT ON THE NERVOUS SYSTEM

During the 1940's it was established that the
clinical effects of DDT are dose-related and involve
the nervous system. Later it was shown that the
degree of dysfunction ranging from mild tremor to
death is related to the concentration of
unmetabolized DDT in the brain at the moment,
regardless of whether illness is produced by one (71)
or many doses (72).

The Biochemical Lesion

Recent discoveries suggest that identification
of the biochemical lesion associated with DDT may be

anticipated. Narahashi and Haas (73) showed by voltage clamp experiments that p,p'-DDT at a concentration of 5 x 10^{-4} moles per liter of bathing medium prolonged Na^+ conductance and reduced K^+ conductance. Matsumura and Patil (74) showed that under certain conditions DDT at concentrations as low as 10^{-8} molar inhibits Na^+, K^+, Mg^{++} -adenosine triphosphatase derived from a nerve ending fraction of the rabbit brain. This enzyme is involved in ion transport in the nervous system. There is a good correlation between the degree of inhibition of this enzyme by analogs of DDT and their toxicity to mosquito larvae. (Incidentally, inhibition of the different ATPase preparation studied by Koch (75) showed no such correlation.)

Both the electrophysiological changes (73) and the enzyme inhibition (74) exhibit a negative temperature coefficient, an important feature of DDT poisoning in insects, probably present in mammals also. It remains to be seen how the enzyme inhibition is related to the electrophysiological changes, particularly since Holan (76) has shown that the toxic action of DDT analogs depends on a critical range of size of the cross-section of the aliphatic side chain of the molecules.

OTHER EFFECTS OF DDT AND ITS ANALOGS

Induction of Microsomal Enzymes

One effect DDT has been shown to share with several drug and other compounds is induction of microsomal enzymes of the liver. To the small extent that this phenomenon has been studied toxicologically, it has been found to be dose-related (77,78). The relatively high dosage received by workers exposed to a number of pesticides (79), or to DDT alone (51), increases the drug metabolizing ability of some workers, with the result that all of them metabolize test drugs with the efficiency found in persons of the general population who are most efficient in this respect. Poland (51) concluded that, because the effect seen in workers is limited, an effect, if any, in the general population must be small.

The threshold dosage of DDT for induction of various microsomal enzymes in the rat has been estimated at about 0.05 mg/kg/day (i.e., a dietary level of 1 ppm) (78) or 0.5 mg/kg/day (80). Datta and Nelson (81) found that a dietary level of 4 ppm (about 0.2 mg/kg/day) induced enzymes. Street (82) estimated the threshold at "1 mg/kg" but presented a figure indicating the threshold may be 0.05 mg/kg/day. The different estimates are not necessarily inconsistent, since they depend on different test systems. In any event, the lowest estimate (0.05 mg/kg/day) is only 0.2 times that known to be effective in man whereas it is 50 times greater than the average dietary intake of all DDT-related materials by a 16- to 19-year-old man, that is 0.0009 mg/kg/day (4).

The enzyme-inducing dosage of 0.5 mg/kg/day used by Schwabe and Wendling (80) led in 14 days to a storage level of 10 ppm in the adipose tissue of rats. The dosage of about 0.2 mg/kg/day used by Datta and Nelson (81) produced in 20 weeks a storage of 39 and 76 ppm in the adipose tissue of males and females, respectively. Twelve weeks after dietary feeding of DDT was stopped, the storage levels of DDT-related materials had fallen to 11 and 21 ppm, respectively, compared to 6 and 9 ppm, respectively, in the controls. The rats previously fed DDT still showed some induction of liver enzymes 12 weeks after dosing was stopped. Neither the rats reported by Schwabe and Wendling nor those reported by Datta and Nelson were in a steady state of DDT storage when their values were between 10 to 21 ppm. It is therefore open to serious question whether these storage values are at all comparable to those found in people in the general population.

Direct Estrogenic Action

DDT, especially o,p'-DDT, has been shown to have an estrogenic effect in rats and birds (83,84). The lowest intraperitoneal dosage producing a significant increase in uterine weight of immature females is 1 mg/kg. The compound is far less efficient than estradiol or diethylstilbesterol, and the minimal effective dosage of the o,p'-isomer is far greater than workers receive as a result of the heaviest occupational exposure.

Action on the Adrenal Cortex and its Secretions

DDD is an insecticide in its own right and a metabolite of DDT. An attempt has been made to use the compound as a drug to control different forms of adrenal overproduction of corticoids in man. The attempt was originally based on the demonstration that DDD (85,86), especially o,p'DDD (87), causes gross atrophy of the adrenals and degeneration of the cells of its inner cortex in dogs. The dosage in human cases has varied from 7 to 285 mg/kg/day, but a dosage of approximately 100 mg/kg/day for many weeks has been necessary to produce any benefit in man (88-94). In contrast, a rate of only 4 mg/kg/day is required to produce marked atrophy of the adrenal in the dog. Kupfer (95) reviewed the extensive literature indicating that the effect in man and other species except the dog is caused by stimulation of corticoid metabolism by massive doses of o,p'-DDD, and not to any direct effect on the adrenal. Southren et al. (91,92) agreed that the effect was predominantly extra-adrenal in man when the drug was first given, but offered evidence that adrenal secretion of cortisol was eventually reduced.

Even large doses of o,p'-DDD cause no histological alteration of the adrenals in man (94). Doses in the therapeutic range, specifically those between 110 and 140 mg/kg/day, produced no detectable injury to the liver, kidney, or bone marrow. All patients treated in this way experienced significant anorexia and nausea, and some showed central nervous system depression varying from lethargy to somnolence. These toxic effects cleared when dosing was discontinued (88).

It has been shown that o,p'-DDD at a concentration of 3×10^{-5} M (10.6 ppm) inhibits lactate dehydrogenase derived from rabbit muscles (96). However, DDD was effective only if added to the reaction mixture before $NADH_2$, a situation unlikely to have a parallel in vivo. Furthermore, p,p'-DDD was as effective as o,p'-DDD, and p,p'-DDT was more effective; thus the degree of inhibition showed no correspondence with effect on the adrenal.

TABLE 3 -- RELATIONSHIP OF DDT DOSAGE TO THE PRODUCTION OF NODULES OR TUMORS IN RODENTS

Species and sex	Dosage (mg/kg/day)		Reference
	Without observed effect	Tumorogenic	
Rat		4.5- 5.3	(100)
Rat, male		≥0.2- 0.7	(97)
Rat, female	2.6	10.5	(97)
Mouse		0.4- 0.7	(101)
Mouse		17.4-46.4	(102)

Tumors

The dosages of DDT reported to have caused nodules or tumors in rodents are summarized in Table 3. Unfortunately, none of the studies was designed to measure the dosage-response relationship of these lesions. Only the work of Ortega et al. (97) permitted the recording of a dosage (2.6 mg/kg/day) that failed to produce nodules in female rats and a higher dosage (10.5 mg/kg/day) that did produce this effect. Investigators have not agreed about the significance of the liver changes they observed in rodents. The chance of reaching a unanimous view is not increased by the fact that the increased susceptibility of protein deficient rats to aflatoxin can be reversed by DDT (98), or by the recent report (99) that about 8% of mice receiving DDT in their diet at a rate of 5.5 mg/kg/day completely resist transplantation of the Zimmerman ependymoma (to which controls are all susceptible), while those in which the tumor becomes established survive significantly longer than control mice receiving no DDT.

Action on Birds

Several species of predatory birds have suffered serious reproductive failure associated with thinning of their eggs, delayed onset of breeding, or both. These changes have been attributed to chlorinated hydrocarbon insecticides, especially DDT or its metabolites through: (a) inhibition of carbonic anhydrase (103,104); (b) excessive metabolism of natural estrogens due to induction of liver microsomal enzymes (104); (c) direct estrogenic action of DDT or its analogs (71); and (d) effect on the thyroid (105). The real importance of these factors or some combination of them in causing the observed population decline is in question. In fact, the same changes have been attributed to polychlorinated biphenyls also (106). Regardless of the mechanism, DDT and its metabolites, especially DDE, almost certainly play a part in thinning the eggshells of susceptible species, for it has been possible to produce the effect experimentally in sparrow hawks (107,108), mallard ducks (109,110), and quail (111). The dosages required were at least as high as those received by DDT factory workers and perhaps higher. However, because of increasing concentrations of DDT and DDE in successive stages of the food chains of susceptible species, the dosages that predatory birds actually may receive in nature are high. Thus the dosages used experimentally are realistic for the species involved, but massive compared to anything people of the general population may receive.

DOSAGES OF DDT TOLERATED BY MAN AND ANIMALS

The dosages absorbed by workers in DDT factories (an average of 0.5 mg/kg/day or less) and tolerated by them without ill effect (50,112) are less than the 10 mg/kg/day tolerated by dogs for over 3 years (113). Rats tolerate 10 mg/kg/day from a clinical standpoint for 2 years, but because of the liver cell changes peculiar to this species, a dosage of 0.25 mg/kg/day is considered the no-effect level in rats (114). In one study, intake of DDT by female rats at the rate of about 2.5 mg/kg/day reduced the number of their young that survived the nursing period, whereas 0.5 mg/kg/day was fully tolerated (115). However, in a later, more complete study, a dietary level of 200 ppm (about 10 mg/kg/day) produced no significant effect on the fecundity of females or the viability of the young (116). The dosages currently absorbed by people in the general population are hundreds of times less than those already tolerated by workers for 20 years -- about one-fourth of their lives. Both the mode of action of DDT and its dosage relationships appear to assure the safety of current levels for people in the general population (see Table 4).

TABLE 4 -- DOSAGE-RESPONSE TO DDT IN MAN

Dosage (mg/kg/day)	Remarks	Reference
?[a]	Fatal	(53)[b]
16-286[a]	Prompt vomiting at higher doses (all poisoned, convulsions in some)	(53)[b]
10[a]	Moderate poisoning in some	(53)[b]
6[a]	Moderate poisoning in one man	(117)
0.5	Tolerated by volunteers for 21 months	(7)
0.5	Tolerated by workers for 6.5 years	(112)
0.25	Tolerated by workers for 19 years	(50)
0.0025	Dosage of general population 1953-4	(6)
0.0004	Current dosage of general population	(4)

[a] One dose only.
[b] Review of many relevant papers.

CONCLUSION

Storage of DDT occurs at the lowest measurable levels of intake. Slight induction of liver microsomal enzymes without detectable clinical effect occurs in men with heavy occupational exposure to DDT. These same workers have not shown other effects of DDT or its analogs whether on the nervous system, the adrenal, the liver, or reproduction. Cases of accidental ingestion make it clear that doses sufficiently higher than those received by workers in a DDT factory will produce typical, acute, neurological poisoning. On the other hand, clinical cases suggest that man is immune to the adrenal atrophy caused by o,p'-DDT in the dog. People are unlikely to experience other effects of DDT because of the large dosages required to produce them and, in some instances, because of species insusceptibility.

The differences in storage of DDT and its analogs among different groups of people (such as formulators, applicators, and the general public) depend on exposure, i.e., dosage. Some differences in the storage of DDT among people living in different countries clearly are caused also by differences in exposure. Whether smaller differences associated with sex, age, or geographical area are partly physiological in origin or whether they are merely secondary to differences in exposure is not known. What must be emphasized is the predominant importance of dosage in determining not only storage but all other effects of DDT.

LEAD

SOURCES OF CONTAMINATION OF THE ENVIRONMENT WITH LEAD AND THEIR SIGNIFICANCE

Lead is present in the environment both as a natural constituent and as a "pollutant." However, current knowledge suggests that clinically evident lead poisoning results only from either industrial or accidental exposure to concentrations of lead which are considerably greater than ambient levels.

Sources of intake of lead in man are the food he eats, the water and other beverages he drinks, and the air he breathes. Of these, food and water are the largest sources of lead for man. The average daily oral intake of lead by adults is roughly 300 micrograms (118). Roughly 10% of this intake is absorbed (119). Inhalation is estimated to contribute an additional 2 to 30 micrograms of lead daily to the intake, the amount depending upon the lead content of the air and the amount of physical activity of the exposed individual.

In the past, poisoning of workers from excess intake of lead due to exposure in lead industries was common. Fortunately, today, clinical lead intoxication in workers is infrequent, except in small, poorly regulated industries such as battery factories or secondary smelters. This improvement is a consequence of strikingly improved practices in industrial medicine. On the other hand, poisoning in children due to ingestion of certain housepaints and in adults from drinking illicitly-distilled whiskeys continues to occur much too frequently.

The toxic effects of lead have been most extensively studied in the hematopoietic (120),

148

neurologic (121), and renal systems (122-125). Other organs of the body such as the heart (126,127) and endocrine glands (128,129) may apparently also be adversely affected but have been less well studied.

The hematopoietic system has received the most investigation (120). The principal abnormality appears to be an interference with heme synthesis. The enzyme delta-aminolevulinic acid dehydrase is particularly sensitive to lead and, according to Hernberg (130), may be inhibited in erythrocytes when the concentration of blood lead is in the range found in individuals exposed to ambient air. As noted previously, it appears that when the blood lead exceeds 40 to 50 µg/100 gm whole blood, the erythropoetic reserve of ALAD of some people is exceeded and the excretion of ALA rises (131). Other effects of lead on the erythropoetic system include impaired uptake of iron by erythroblasts and shortening of the red cell survival.

Nervous system manifestations of plumbism include peripheral neuropathy, myelopathy and injury to the cerebral cortex (132). Damage to the cerebrum may result from acute encephalopathy, or possibly from chronic exposure to lower concentrations for long periods of time. The myelopathy is relatively rare while the peripheral neuropathy is common. Recent observations by Catton et al. (121) suggest that effects of lead on peripheral nerves may occur in some individuals exposed to relatively low levels of lead such as occur in certain modern industries.

Damage to kidneys also occurs as a consequence of severe lead intoxication (122-125). The renal tubule appears particularly sensitive to injury and prolonged exposure may lead to renal failure. It is considered doubtful that current levels of occupational exposure in well regulated industries are hazardous in this respect (122).

BODY STORES OF LEAD

Under steady state conditions, more than 90% of the lead in the body is in the skeleton. This lead has traditionally been considered sequestered and non-toxic. However, bone is not inert. Since it actively turns over calcium and other minerals, it is to be expected that an unknown quantity of lead in bone may be released to soft tissues under proper circumstances. Conditions such as acidosis, fractures, or immobilization may cause lead to be released even more rapidly and conceivably may sometimes cause toxicity (119). Post-mortem analysis indicates the lead concentration in bone and aorta increases with age (133,134).

The accumulation of lead in the soft tissues where it inhibits crucial enzymes is responsible for the toxic effects of this metal (135). Greatest concentrations are found in the liver, aorta, and kidney with lesser amounts in the muscle and brain (119).

In measuring the body burden of lead, most attention has been paid to the levels in blood and urine (Table 1). There appears to be little question that the values obtained from blood appear to be a reasonable index of the lead content of soft tissue if the hematocrit is near normal. The major advantage of blood over urine includes the convenience of collection and the fact that nearly all the lead in blood is bound to erythrocytes. The body burden of lead may also be assessed by measuring the urinary lead excretion following administration of chelating agents such as calcium disodium ethylene diamine tetraacetate (Ca-Na$_2$EDTA) (136,137). This

TABLE 5 -- CONCENTRATIONS OF LEAD IN BLOOD OF SELECTED GROUPS OF MEN[a]

Mean Lead Concentration in Blood (mg/100g)	Number of Subjects	Group
0.012	16	Residents of rural California county
0.013	10	Commuter nonsmokers, Philadelphia
0.015	15	Suburban smokers, Philadelphia
0.021	33	Commuter smokers, Philadelphia
0.021	155	Policemen, Los Angeles
0.022	11	Live and work downtown, non-smokers, Philadelphia
0.024	30	Policemen, nonsmokers, Philadelphia
0.026	83	Policemen, smokers, Philadelphia
0.028	130	Service station attendants, Cincinnati
0.030	40	Traffic policemen, Cincinnati
0.030	60	Tunnel employees, Boston
0.031	14	Drivers of cars, Cincinnati
0.034	48	Parking lot attendants, Cincinnati

[a] Adapted from Three Cities Study (138).

technique is particularly useful in individuals who have had intermittent exposure to lead, and who are not currently in a high lead environment. The measurement of lead in hair may offer a potentially useful technique but requires further evaluation before it can be applied.

Hammond (119) has reported on the results of a survey conducted in 1961-62 of the lead concentration in the urine and blood of individuals in three large metropolitan areas. These studies, conducted under the auspices of the U. S. Public Health Service, were compared with earlier studies to see if any trends in concentration of lead in these two fluids were evident. The results of these studies indicated:

a. The concentration of lead in the blood and urine of these urban dwellers had not increased over the level found during the previous five years.

b. The concentration of lead in the blood and urine increased in proportion to involvement with conditions of high automobile traffic density.

c. There was no evidence that the concentration of lead in the blood or urine increased with age.

REFERENCES

1. Dale, W. E. and Quinby, G. E. (1963). Chlorinated insecticides in the body fat of people in the United States. Science 142: 593.

2. Dale, W. E., Copeland, M. F. and Hayes, W. J. (1965). Chlorinated insecticides in the body fat of people in India. Bull. WHO 33: 471.

3. Hayes, W. J. (1966). Monitoring food and people for pesticide content. Scientific aspects of pest control. National Research Council symposium, Washington, D. C. NAS-NRC Publ. No. 1402: 314.

4. Duggan, R. E. (1968). Residues in food and feed. Pesticide residue levels in foods in the United States from July 1, 1963, to June 30, 1967. Pest. Monit. J. 2: 2.

5. Durham, W. F., Armstrong, J. F. and Quinby, G. E. (1965). DDT and DDE content of complete prepared meals. Arch. Env. Health 11: 641.

6. Walker, K. C., Goette, M. B., and Batchelor, G. S. (1954). Pesticide residues in foods. Dichloro diphenyl trichloroethane and dichloro diphenyl dichloroethylene content of prepared meals. J. Agric. Food Chem. 2: 1034.

7. Hayes, W. J., Dale, W. E. and Pirkle, C. I. (1971). Evidence of safety of long-term, high, oral doses of DDT for man. Arch. Env. Health 22: 119.

8. Davies, J. E., Welke, J. O. and Radomski, J. L. (1965). Epidemiological aspects of the use of pesticides in the South. J. Occup. Med. 7: 612.

9. Davies, J. E. et al. (1968). Problems of prevalence of pesticide residues in humans. Pest. Monit. J. 2: 80.

10. Hayes, W. J., Durham, W. F. and Cueto, C. (1956). The effect of known repeated oral doses of chlorophenothane (DDT) in man. J. Amer. Med. Assoc. 162: 890.

11. Hayes, W. J. et al. (1958). Storage of DDT and DDE in people with different degrees of exposure to DDT. Amer. Med. Assoc. Arch. Indust. Health 18: 398.

12. Hayes, W. J., Dale, W. E. and Burse, V. W. (1965). Chlorinated hydrocarbon pesticides in the fat of people in New Orleans. Life Sci. 4: 1611.

13. Hoffman, W. S., Fishbein, W. I. and Andelman, M. B. (1964). The pesticide content of human fat tissue. Arch. Env. Health 9: 387.

14. Hoffman, W. S., Adler, H. and Fishbein, W. I. (1967). Relation of pesticide concentrations in fat to pathological changes in tissues. Arch. Env. Health 15: 758.

15. Laug, E. P., Kunze, F. M. and Prickett, C. S. (1951). Occurrence of DDT in human fat and milk. Arch. Indust. Hyg. Occup. Med. 3: 245.

16. Quinby, G. E. et al. (1965). DDT storage in the U. S. populations. J. Amer. Med. Assoc. 191: 175.

17. Radomski, J. L. et al. (1968). Pesticide concentrations in the liver, brain, and adipose tissue of terminal hospital patients. Food Cosmet. Toxicol. 6: 209.

18. Schafer, M. L. and Campbell, J. E. (1966). Distribution of pesticide residues in human body tissues from Montgomery County, Ohio. In: R. F. Gould, (ed.), Organic Pesticides in the Environment. Advances in Chemistry Series # 60, American Chemical Society, Washington, D. C., 89.

19. Zavon, M. R., Hine, C. H. and Parker, K. D. (1965). Chlorinated hydrocarbon insecticides in human body fat in the United States. J. Amer. Med. Assoc. 193: 837.

20. Brown, J. R. (1967). Organo-chlorine pesticide residues in human depot fat. Can. Med. Assoc. J. 97: 367.

21. Read, S. I. and McKinley, W. P. (1961). DDT and DDE content of human fat. A survey. Arch. Env. Health 3: 209.

22. Casarett, L. J. et al. (1968). Organochlorine pesticide residues in human tissue - Hawaii. Arch. Env. Health 17: 306.

23. Fiserova-Bergerova, V. et al. (1967). Levels of chlorinated hydrocarbon pesticides in human tissues. Indust. Med. Surg. 36: 65.

24. Dale, W. E. (1971). Personal communication.

25. Maes, R. and Heyndrickx, A. (1966). Distribution of organic chlorinated insecticides in human tissues. Meded. Rijksfaculteit Landbouwwetenschappen Gent. 31: 1021.

26. Halačka, H., Hakl, J. and Vymětal, F. (1965). Effect of massive doses of DDT on human adipose tissue. Cesk. Hyg. 10: 188.

27. Weihe, M. (1966). Chlorinated insecticides in the body fat of people in Denmark. Ugeskrift Laeger 128: 881.

28. Abbott, D. C., Goulding, R. and Tatton, J. O'G. (1968). Organochlorine pesticide residues in human fat in Great Britain. Brit. Med. J. 3: 146.

29. Cassidy, W. et al. (1967). Organo-chlorine pesticide residues in human fats from Somerset. Monthly Bull. Minist. Health Lab. Serv. 26: 2.

30. Egan, H. et al. (1965). Organo-chlorine pesticide residues in human fat and human milk. Brit. Med. J. 2: 66.

31. Hunter, C. G., Robinson, J. and Richardson, A. (1963). Chlorinated insecticide content of human body fat in Southern England. Brit. Med. J. 1: 221.

32. Robinson, J. and Hunter, C. G. (1966). Organochlorine insecticides: Concentrations in human blood and adipose tissue. Arch. Env. Health 13: 558.

33. Hayes, W. J., Dale, W. E. and LeBreton, R. (1963). Storage of insecticides in French people. Nature 199: 1189.

34. Engst, R., Knoll, R. and Nickel, B. (1967). Über die Anreicherung von chlorierten Kohlenwasserstoffen, insbesondere von DDT und seinem metaboliten DDE, in menschlichen Fett. Pharmazie 22: 654.

35. Maier-Bode, H. (1960). DDT in human body fat. Med. Exptl. 1: 148.

36. Denés, A. (1962). Lebensmittelchemische Probleme von Rückstanden chlorierter Kohlenwasserstoffe. Nahrung 6: 48.

37. Kanitz, S. and Castello, G. (1966). Sulla presenza di residui di alcuni disinfestanti nel tessuto adiposo umano ed in alcuni alimenti. Giornals di Igene e Medicina Preventiva 7: 1.

38. de Vlieger, M. et al. (1968). The organochlorine insecticide content of human tissues. Arch. Env. Health 17: 759.

39. Wit, S. L. (1964). Aspects of toxicology and chemical analysis of insecticide residues. Voeding 25: 609.

40. Bronisz, H. et al. (1967). DDT in adipose tissue of Polish population. Diss. Pharm. Pharmakol. 19: 309.

41. Aizicovici, et al. (1966). Travaux Scientifiques de l'Institut d'Hygiene de Jassy, 1960-1966, 142. (Cited by Crede, Wassermann, M. et al. (1968). Proc. Lagos International Seminar on Occupational Health for Developing Countries, Nigeria.)

42. Llinares, V. M. and Wasserman, M. (1967). Storage of DDT in the body fat of people in Spain. 2nd Nat. Congr. Med. Agricola, Valencia. (Cited by Crede, Wassermann, M. et al. (1968) Proc. Lagos International Seminar on Occupational Health for Developing Countries, Nigeria.)

43. Wassermann, M. et al. (1965). DDT and DDE in the body fat of the people of Israel. Arch. Env. Health 11: 375.

44. Wassermann, M. et al. (1967). Storage of DDT in the people of Israel. Pest. Monit. J. 1: 15.

45. Wassermann, M. et al. (1968). Storage of organochlorine insecticides in body fat of people in Nigeria. Proc. Lagos International Seminar on Occupational Health for Developing Countries, Nigeria.

46. Bick, M. (1967). Chlorinated hydrocarbon residues in human fat. Med. J. Australia 1: 1127.

47. Wassermann, M. et al. (1968). Storage of organochlorine pesticides in the body fat of people in Western Australia. Indust. Med. Surg. 37: 295.

48. Brewerton, K. V. and McGrath, H. J. W. (1967). Insecticides in human fat in New Zealand. New Zeal. J. Sci. Technol. 10: 486.

49. Durham, W. F. et al. (1961). Insecticide content of diet and body fat of Alaskan natives. Science 134: 1880.

50. Laws, E. R., Curley, A. and Biros, F. J. (1967). Men with intensive occupational exposure to DDT. A clinical and chemical study. Arch. Env. Health 15: 766.

51. Poland, A. et al. (1970). Effect of intensive occupational exposure to DDT on phenylbutazone and crotisol metabolism in human subjects. Clin. Pharmacol. Therap. 11: 724.

52. Mattson, A. M. et al. (1953). Determination of DDT and related substances in human fat. Anal. Chem. 25: 1065.

53. Hayes, W. J. (1959). Pharmacology and toxicology of DDT. In: Paul Muller, (ed.), DDT, The Insecticide Dichlorodiphenyl-trichloroethane and its Significance. Birkhäuser, Verlag, Basel, II: 9.

54. Dale, W. E., Curley, A. and Cueto, C. (1966). Hexane extractable chlorinated insecticides in human blood. Life Sci. 5: 47.

55. Radomski, J. L. and Fiserova-Bergerova, V. (1965). The determination of pesticides in tissues with the electron capture detector without prior clean-up. Indust. Med. Surg. 34: 934.

56. Neal, P. A. et al. (1946). The excretion of DDT (2,2-bis-[p-chlorophenyl]-1,1,1-trichloroethane) in man, together with clinical observations. U. S. Public Health Rpts. 61: 403.

57. Durham, W. F., Armstrong, J. F. and Quinby, G. E. (1965). DDA excretion levels. Arch. Env. Health 11: 76.

58. Cueto, C. and Biros, F. J. (1967). Chlorinated insecticides and related materials in human urine. Toxicol. Appl. Pharmacol. 10: 261.

59. Cranmer, M. F., Carroll, J. J. and Copeland, M. F. (1969). Determination of DDT and metabolites, including DDA, in human urine by gas chromatography. Bull. Env. Contam. Toxicol. 4: 214.

60. Quinby, G. E., Armstrong, J. F. and Durham, W. F. (1965). DDT in human milk. Nature 207: 726.

61. West, I. (1964). Pesticides as contaminants. Arch. Env. Health 9: 626.

62. Curley, A. and Kimbrough, R. D. (1969). Chlorinated hydrocarbon insecticides in plasma and milk of pregnant and lactating women. Arch. Env. Health 18: 156.

63. Denés, A. (1964). Investigation of chlorinated hydrocarbon residues in animal and vegetable fats. In: 1963 Year-Book Inst. Nutr., Budapest, 46.

64. Damaskin, V. I. (1965). The extent of the accumulation of DDT in the human body in connection with its assimilation with food, and its toxic effects. Gig. i. Sanit. 30: 109.

65. Bronisz, H. and Ochynski, J. (1968). DDT and DDE in human milk. Biuletyn Instytutu Ochrony Roslin 41: 99.

66. Lofroth, G. (1968). Pesticides and catastrophe. New Scientist 40: 567.

67. Gracheva, G. V. (1969). The possibility of DDT accumulation in the organism of persons not having occupational contact with it. Faktory Vneshn. Sredy i ikh Znachen 1: 125.

68. Heyndrickx, A. and Maes, R. (1969). The excretion of chlorinated hydrocarbon insecticides in human mother milk. J. Pharmacol. Belg. 9-10: 459.

69. Hruska, J. (1969). DDT residues in the milk, butter, and fat of cattle. Veterinarstvi 19: 493.

70. Komarova, L. I. (1970). The excretion of DDT in mother's milk and its effect on the organism of mother and child. Pediatrija, Akuserstvo I Ginekologija 1.

71. Dale, W. E. et al. (1963). Poisoning by DDT: Relation between clinical signs and concentration in rat brain. Science 142: 1474.

72. Hayes, W. J. and Dale, W. E. (1964). Concentration of DDT in brain and other tissues in relation to symptomatology. Toxicol. Appl. Pharmacol. 6: 349.

73. Narahashi, T. and Haas, H. G. (1967). DDT: Interaction with nerve membrane conductance changes. Science 157: 1438.

74. Matsumura, F. and Patil, K. C. (1969). Adenosine triphosphatase sensitive to DDT in synapses of rat brain. Science 166: 121.

75. Koch, R. B. (1969). Chlorinated hydrocarbon insecticides: Inhibition of rabbit brain ATPase activities. J. Neurochem. 16: 269.

76. Holan, G. (1971). Rational design of insecticides. Bull. WHO 44: 355.

77. Durham, W. F. (1967). The interaction of pesticides with other factors. Residue Rev. 18: 21.

78. Kinoshita, F. K., Frawley, J. P. and DuBois, K. P. (1966). Quantitative measurement of induction of hepatic microsomal enzymes by various dietary levels of DDT and toxaphene in rats. Toxicol. Appl. Pharmacol. 9: 505.

79. Kolmodin, B., Azarnoff, D. L. and Sjoqvist, F. (1969). Effect of environmental factors on drug metabolism: Decreased plasma half-life of antipyrine in workers exposed to chlorinated hydrocarbon insecticides. Clin. Pharmacol. Therap. 10: 638.

80. Schwabe, U. and Wendling, I. (1967). Beschleunigung des Arzneimittel-abbaus durch kleine Dosen von DDT und anderen chlorkohlenwasserstoff-Insekticiden. Arzneimittel Forsch. 17: 614.

81. Datta, P. R. and Nelson, M. J. (1968). Enhanced metabolism of methyprylon, meprobamate, and chlordiazepoxide hydrochloride after chronic feeding of a low dietary level of DDT to male and female rats. Toxicol. Appl. Pharmacol. 13: 346.

82. Street, J. C. (1968). Modification of animal responses to toxicants. In: E. Hodgson, (ed.), The Enzymatic Oxidation of Toxicants. Proc. Conf. North Carolina State University, Raleigh, North Carolina, 197.

83. Bitman, J. et al. (1968). Estrogenic activity of o,p'-DDT in the mammalian uterus and avian oviduct. Science 162: 371.

84. Welch, R. M., Levin, W. and Conney, A. H. (1969). Estrogenic action of DDT and its analogs. Toxicol. Appl. Pharmacol. 14: 358.

85. Nelson, A. A. and Woodard, G. (1948). Adrenal cortical atrophy and liver damage produced in dogs by feeding 2,2-bis-(parachlorophenyl) 1,1-dichloroethane (DDD). Fed. Proc. 7: 277.

86. Nelson, A. A. and Woodard, G. (1949). Several adrenal cortical atrophy (cytotoxic) and hepatic damage produced in dogs by feeding

2,2-bis(parachlorophenyl)-1,1-dichloroethane
(DDD or TDE). Arch. Path. 48: 387.

87. Cueto, C. and Brown, J. H. U. (1962).
Biological studies on an adrenocorticolytic
agent and the isolation of the active
components. Endocrinology 62: 334.

88. Bergenstal, D. M. et al. (1960). Chemotherapy
of adrenocortical cancer with o,p'-DDD. Ann.
Int. Med. 53: 672.

89. Bledsoe, T. et al. (1964). An effect of
o,p'-DDD on the extra-adrenal metabolism of
cortisol in man. J. Clin. Endocrinol. 24:
1303.

90. Gallagher, T. F., Fukushima, D. K. and Hellman,
L. (1962). The effect of ortho, para'DDD on
steroid hormone metabolites in adrenocortical
carcinoma. Met. Clin. Exp. 11: 1155.

91. Southren, A. L. et al. (1966). The effect of
2,2-bis(2-chlorophenyl-4-chlorophenyl)
-1,1-dichloroethane(o,p'-DDD) on the
metabolism of infused cortisol-7-^{3}H.
Steroids 7: 11.

92. Southren, A. L. et al. (1966). Remission in
Cushing's syndrome with o,p'-DDD. J. Clin.
Endocrinol. Metab. 26: 268.

93. Verdon, T. A. et al. (1962). Clinical and
chemical response of functioning adrenal
cortical carcinoma to o,p'-DDD. Metabolism 11:
226.

94. Wallace, Z. E. et al. (1961). Cushing's
syndrome due to adrenocortical hyperplasia.
New Eng. J. Med. 265: 1088.

95. Kupfer, D. (1967). Effects of some pesticides
and related compounds on steroid function and
metabolism. Residue Rev. 19: 11.

96. Cazorla, A. (1964). Inhibition of lactate
dehydrogenase by DDT and other related
substances. Biochim. Biophys. Acta 81: 593.

97. Ortega, P. et al. (1956). DDT in the diet of the rat. Public Health Monogr. 43, Public Health Serv. Publ. 484.

98. McLean, A. E. M. and McLean, E. K. (1969). Diet and toxicity. Brit. Med. Bull. 25: 278.

99. Laws, E. R. (1971). Evidence of antitumorogenic effects of DDT. Arch. Env. Health 23: 181.

100. Fitzhugh, O. G. and Nelson, A. A. (1947). The chronic oral toxicity of DDT 2,2-bis[(p-chlorophenyl-1,1,1-trichloroethane)]. J. Pharmacol. Exptl. Therap. 89: 18.

101. Tarján, R. and Kemény, T. (1969). Multigeneration studies on DDT in mice. Food Cosmet. Toxicol. 7: 215.

102. Innes, J. R. M. et al. (1969). Bioassay of pesticides and industrial chemicals for tumorigenicity in mice. A preliminary note. J. Nat. Cancer Inst. 42: 1101.

103. Bitman, J., Cecil, H. C. and Fries, G. F. (1970). DDT-induced inhibition of avian shell gland carbonic anhydrase: A mechanism for thin eggshells. Science 168: 594.

104. Peakall, D. B. (1970). Pesticides and the reproduction of birds. Sci. Amer. 222: 72.

105. Jefferies, D. J. and French, M. C. (1969). Avian thyroid: Effect of p,p'-DDT on size and activity. Science 166: 1278.

106. Risebrough, R. W. et al. (1968). Polychlorinated biphenyls in the global ecosystem. Nature 220: 1098.

107. Porter, R. D. and Wiemeyer, S. N. (1969). Dieldrin and DDT: Effects on sparrow hawk eggshells and reproduction. Science 165: 199.

108. Wiemeyer, S. N. and Porter, R. D. (1970). DDE thins eggshells of captive American kestrels. Nature 227: 737.

109. Heath, R. G., Spann, J. W. and Kreitzer, J. F. (1969). Marked DDE impairment of mallard reproduction in controlled studies. Nature 224: 47.

110. Tucker, R. K. and Haegele, H. A. (1970). Eggshell thinning as influenced by method of DDT exposure. Bull. Environ. Contamin. Toxicol. 5: 191.

111. Bitman, J. et al. (1969). DDT induces a decrease in eggshell calcium. Nature 224: 44.

112. Ortelee, M. F. (1958). Study of men with prolonged intensive occupational exposure to DDT. Arch. Indust. Health 18: 433.

113. Lehman, A. J. (1952). Chemicals in foods: A report to the Association of Food and Drug Officials on current developments. Part II. Pesticides; Sec. III. Subacute and chronic toxicity. Assoc. Food Drug Off. Quart. Bull. XVI, 47.

114. Lehman, A. J. (1965). Summaries of pesticide toxicity. Assoc. Food Drug Off. United States, Topeka, Kansas.

115. Fitzhugh, O. G. (1948). Use of DDT insecticides on food products. Indust. Eng. Chem. 40: 704.

116. Ottoboni, A. (1969). Effect of DDT on reproduction in the rat. Toxicol. Appl. Pharmacol. 14: 74.

117. Hsieh, H. C. (1954). DDT intoxication in a family in Southern Taiwan. Arch. Indust. Hyg. 10: 344.

118. Cholak, J. and Bomback, K. (1943). Measurement of industrial lead exposure by analysis of blood and excreta of workmen. J. Indust. Hyg. Toxicol. 25: 47.

119. Hammond, P. B. (1969). Lead poisoning, an old problem with a new dimension. In F. R. Blood, (ed.), Essays in Toxicology. I. Academic Press, New York, 116.

120. Griggs, R. C. (1964). Lead poisoning: hematologic aspects. In: C. V. Moore and E. B. Brown, (eds.), Progress in Hematology. Grune and Stratton, Inc., New York, IV: 117.

121. Catton, M. J. et al. (1970). Sub-clinical neuropathy in lead workers. Brit. Med. J. 2: 80.

122. Black, D. A. K. (1965). Metals and the kidney. Ann. Occup. Hyg. 8: 17.

123. Chisholm, J. J. (1962). Amino aciduria as a manifestation of renal tubular injury in lead intoxication and a comparison with patterns of amino aciduria seen in other diseases. J. Pediatr. 60: 1.

124. Emmerson, B. T. (1963). Chronic lead nephropathy. Aust. Ann. Med. 12: 310.

125. Goyer, R. A. (1968). The renal tubule in lead poisoning. I. Mitochondrial swelling and amino aciduria. Lab Invest. 19: 71.

126. Myerson, R. M. and Eisenhauer, J. H. (1963). Atrioventricular conduction defects in lead poisoning. Amer. J. Cardiol. 11: 409.

127. Silver, W. and Rodrigues-Torres, R. (1968). Electrocardiographic studies in children with lead poisoning. Pediatrics 41: 1124.

128. McAllister, R. G., Michelakis, A. M. and Sandstead, H. H. (1971). Plasma renin activity in chronic plumbism. Effect of treatment. Arch. Int. Med. 127: 919.

129. Sandstead, H. H., Stant, E. G. and Brill, A. B. (1969). Lead intoxication and the thyroid. Arch. Int. Med. 123: 632.

130. Hernberg, S. et al. (1970). Delta-aminolevulinic acid dehydrase as a measure of lead poisoning. Arch. Env. Health 21: 140.

131. Selander, S. and Cramer, K. (1970). Interrelationships between lead in blood, lead in urine, and ALA in urine during lead work. Brit. J. Indust. Med. 27: 28.

132. Simpson, J. A., Seaton, D. A. and Adams, J. F. (1964). Response to treatment with chelating agents of anemia, chronic encephalopathy, and myelopathy due to lead poisoning. J. Neurol. Neurosurg. Psychiat. 27: 536.

133. Horiuchi, K., Horiguchi, S. and Suekane, M. (1959). Studies on industrial lead poisoning. Absorption, transportation, deposition, and excretion of lead. The lead contents in organic tissues of the normal Japanese. Osaka City Med. J. 5: 41.

134. Schroeder, H. A. and Tipton, I. L. H. (1968). The human body burden of lead. Arch. Env. Health 17: 965.

135. Ulmer, D. D. and Vallee, B. L. (1969). Effects of lead on biochemical systems. In: D. D. Hemphill, (ed.), Trace Substances in Environmental Health II. University of Missouri Press, Columbia, Missouri, 7.

136. Přerovská, I. and Teisinger, J. (1970). Excretion of lead and its biological activity several years after termination of exposure. Brit. J. Ind. Med. 27: 352.

137. Teisinger, J. and Srbova, J. (1958). The value of mobilization of lead by calcium ethylene diamine tetra acetate in the diagnosis of lead poisoning. Brit. J. Indust. Med. 16: 148.

138. Cincinnati: Division of Air Pollution, Public Health Service, U. S. Dept. Health, Education, and Welfare. (1965). Survey of Lead in the Atmosphere of Three Urban Communities. Public Health Serv. Publ. No. 999-AP-12, 94 pp.

CHAPTER 11. BODY BURDENS
OF RADIOACTIVITY

A. B. BRILL, F. L. PARKER, and R. E. JOHNSTON
Vanderbilt University, Nashville, Tennessee

More effort has been devoted to the study of
ionizing radiations and their potential hazard to man
than any other single agent or group of agents.
These unusual radiations have been viewed as
fundamentally interesting phenomena worthy of study
from the time of their first discovery. Wide ranging
applications and concern regarding potential hazards
has led to a great investment of time and effort on
the part of scientists, engineers, and physicians and
much information of fundamental importance has
resulted from these studies. The development and
dissemination of nuclear power sources (reactors)
have contributed to the exposures of persons in the
immediate environs and have been the subject
of popular and scientific debate. The benefits in
terms of continued availability and cost of
power so produced are tangible, and society is in
the process of weighing these against the merits
and hazards of alternative power sources. The number
and kind of radioactive materials used in medicine
have increased rapidly in recent years and
provide significant benefit to patients. The
doses in therapy are many fold higher than for
diagnostic studies, which are in turn many fold
greater than those received from other man-made
and naturally-occurring radioisotopic sources.
The number of persons exposed medically is small, in
contrast to the large population exposed to smaller
environmental doses from fallout or power
reactors.

Various national and international committees
have reviewed and summarized the extensive

information relating to radioactive isotope exposures and hazards. The reports of the United National Scientific Committee on the Effects of Atomic Radiation summarize and clearly document the current state of knowledge on this topic (1-5).

NATURALLY OCCURRING RADIOACTIVE NUCLIDES

RADIOACTIVITY IN THE EARTH'S CRUST -- Naturally occurring radioactive materials are widely distributed throughout the earth's crust and contribute to mankind's radiation exposure from a value somewhat less than that due to cosmic rays (50 mrem/year GSD on the average) to values in some regions which are many times greater (Table 1). The major sources of radioactivity in the earth's crust are uranium-238, thorium-232, radium-226, and their daughter products, along with potassium-40 and cosmic ray produced radioisotopes of carbon and hydrogen. Many other radioactive materials exist but in low abundance and of negligible consequence.

With the exception of certain areas in the world where radionuclide concentrations are unusually high (monazite sands), the mean dose rate to the gonads and bone received by the world population from external exposure to terrestrial gamma radiation is about 47 mrads/year. Persons living in certain granite-rich areas of France receive mean gonadal

TABLE 1 -- EXPOSURE OF MAN TO NATURALLY OCCURRING RADIONUCLIDES (5)

Type of Exposure	Mean Dose to Gonads mrad/yr	Mean Dose to Bone mrad/yr	Mean Dose to Lungs mrad/yr
Internal			
^{40}K	18 - 22	7 - 11	15
^{226}Ra + daughter products		3 - 7	0.5
^{14}C	0.7 - 1.8	1.5	
^{220}, ^{222}Rn wooden house			45
brick house			104
concrete house			158
External			
Normal Regions	47		
Granite Regions in France	162	(approximately the same	
Monazite Regions in India	802	as for gonads)	
Monazite Regions in Brazil	287		

Total for normal regions (GSD) = 69 mrem/yr.

doses of 162 mrads/year, while persons living on monazite sands in Brazil and Karala, India, are exposed respectively to 287 and 802 mrads/year on the average. In addition, the lung is exposed to radon-220 and radon-222 released from different building materials. Living in a wooden house results in a lung exposure of approximately 45 mrads/year as opposed to 104 mrads/year from brick houses, and 158 mrads/year from concrete houses on the average (6). No evidence currently available shows disease gradients which can be related to levels of background radiation exposure.

RADIOACTIVITY IN FOOD AND WATER -- Drinking water and food contain variable amounts of radioactive material of natural origin which may be retained in the body after ingestion. Elements of the uranium and thorium series, potassium-40 and carbon-14 are the main natural sources of radioactivity deposited in the body. Potassium and carbon are distributed throughout the whole body and hence contribute to the gonadal as well as to the bone dose. Radium taken internally through food and water contributes primarily to bone dose. The mean dose to the gonads from these internal exposures is between 19 and 24 mrads/year. The mean dose to the bone is between 12 and 24 mrads/year, the average value being about 16, and comes primarily from potassium-40 and not from radium as might have been expected. The dose received by the lung tissue is derived in part from potassium-40 but mostly from the radon-daughters of radium from dietary sources. For normal regions, the mean dose to the gonads from naturally occurring radionuclides is 69 mrem/year, which is 38.5% of the genetically significant dose (GSD) estimated for the U.S.A. (6).

IRRADIATION FROM RADIOACTIVE CONTAMINATION OF THE ENVIRONMENT DUE TO EXPLOSIONS OF NUCLEAR WEAPONS

Considerable data are available in the literature concerning the contamination of the environment with radioactivity resulting from nuclear weapons testing (Table 2). Since almost all atmospheric weapons testing ceased in 1962, fall-out now represents a proportionally small contribution to population exposure.

TABLE 2 -- DOSE COMMITMENTS (mrad) FROM NUCLEAR TESTS
CARRIED OUT BEFORE 1968 (5)

Source of Radiation	Tissue			
	Gonads	Cells Lining Bone Surfaces	Bone Marrow	Thyroid of 0-1 year old
External	46	46	46	46
Internal				
^{90}Sr	--	130	64	--
^{137}Cs	21	21	21	21
^{14}C	13	16	13	13
^{131}I	--	--	--	330
Total to Year 2000	80	213	144	410
Avg. dose rate/ year	1.7	4.6	3.1	8.9
Dose from ^{14}C after year 2000 (7)	167	270	167	167

The major sources of external exposures from fall-out are from the short-lived gamma-emitting radionuclides, zirconium-95, niobium-95, and the longer-lived cesium-137. The tissue dose delivered from deposited fall-out not incorporated into the body depends upon the shielding effect of buildings, the fraction of time individuals spend outdoors, and the rate at which the radioactive debris settles onto the land.

Internal exposure is primarily from strontium-90, cesium-137, iodine-131, and carbon-14 (Table 2). Diet, including both plant and animal foods, is the principal source of intake. The distribution of strontium in the body follows closely that of calcium. It is, therefore, deposited in the skeleton and retained for a period of years. The beta radiation from strontium-90 irradiates not only the bone itself, but also the bone-forming and blood-forming cells contained in the bone cavities. Cesium-137 is uniformly distributed throughout the body and has a considerably shorter biological half-life than strontium-90.

The explosion of nuclear weapons has added considerably to the amount of naturally-occurring cosmic ray produced carbon-14 in the atmosphere. By 1959, there was an increase of about 30% above background (2) and, by 1963, carbon-14 levels had increased by 80% over pre-1952 values (7). The dose rate from carbon-14 is small compared to that from other radionuclides produced by nuclear explosions. Carbon-14, because of its very long residence time in the biosphere, and its 5,760 year radioactive half-life, will continue to contaminate the environment for thousands of years to come. This constitutes a potential genetic hazard because of the many generations which will be exposed to this radionuclide.

Iodine-131 is produced in relatively high yields by atomic explosions. It is short-lived (8-day physical half-life) but selectively concentrates in the thyroid gland. It is secreted in milk and reaches the body by ingestion of fresh foods, milk being the principal source. The dose to the thyroid from uptake of iodine-131 varies with age. Because of the small size of the gland in infancy and the high milk consumption in this age group, the maximum dose rate from iodine-131 contamination of the environment occurs in the 0 to 1 year age group.

The accumulated dose in mrads from past nuclear weapons testing and extrapolations to the year 2000 and beyond is shown towards the bottom of Table 2. Assuming no further weapons testing, and based upon the measured dose rates from fall-out during the period from 1954 to 1962, the average gonadal dose rate is 1.7 mrads/year, and the average bone dose rate is between 3 and 5 mrads/year. The largest dose commitments are received from strontium-90 by the cells lining the bone surfaces and from iodine-131 by the thyroid during the first year of life. The integral dose from carbon-14 after year 2000 is greater than that from all other fall-out products with the exception of the thyroid dose from iodine-131.

The cumulative radiation dose received by the bone marrow from natural background during the year 1954-2000 is shown as the hatched portion of Fig. 1 on top of which is added the dose commitment received during the same number of years from fall-out due to weapons testing during the years up to 1962. This shows the fall-out contribution to an average individual born in 1954. Individuals born before or

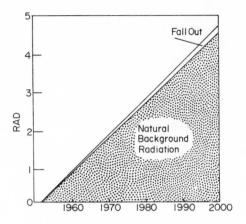

Fig. 1. Contributions of dose commitment to bone marrow from natural background and fall out to the year 2000 (8).

after this date on the average receive a smaller proportion of their total exposure from fall-out. The increment in average population exposure from fall-out from weapons testing is not impressive when compared to that received from natural background radiation. However, concentration mechanisms in the environment can cause much higher doses to individuals. For example, cesium-137 deposited on Arctic lichens builds up over the years and is a major contaminant of reindeer food. Consequently, reindeer meat has a high concentration of cesium-137 and those who have a large component of reindeer meat in their diet do receive larger than average whole body dosages.

NUCLEAR POWER PLANTS AND THE ATOMIC ENERGY INDUSTRY

Assessment of population exposures from the use of reactors for the production of nuclear power depends upon the amount of nuclear power generated, the type of plants used, waste management practices, and the population density in the immediate and more remote environs. In 1969, the U. S. Atomic Energy Commission's forecast for the growth of nuclear power estimated a 1 million megawatt nuclear power capacity (9) for the United States by the year 2000, which is assumed to be 25% of the world total nuclear power production in that year (10). Assuming the same

170

types of reactors are used through the rest of this century, and the operating experience of the thirteen nuclear power plants in the U. S. in 1969, average population exposures can be computed.

The A.E.C. standard that has governed reactor releases is 500 mrem/yr to individuals at a point in space, namely the site boundary. A.E.C. has proposed that this be reduced to 5 mrem/yr from materials in liquid effluents and 5 mrem/yr from radioactive material in gaseous effluents for light water reactors (11). The dose at the reactor site boundary diminishes with distance from the boundary, by dispersion and decay, so that Bond estimates that at 50 miles the dose is about one-tenth of one percent of that at the site boundary (12). Figures determined from experience with currently operating power reactors reveals doses of about 5 mrem and .005 mrem/yr, respectively, at the site boundary and at 50 miles (13). The average dose from these sources to people within a 50-mile radius of these reactors is approximately 0.01 mrem/yr (13).

Parker has taken the data on current reactor practices and the anticipated growth of the nuclear power industry and has computed the expected doses from nuclear power plants in the year 2000 (14). These are presented in Table 3.

The highest per capita doses are estimated for Europe and the U. S. A. with per capita values expected to lie between 1 and 3 mrem/yr assuming that reactors will generate 4 million megawatts of power, i.e. an approximately four-hundred fold increase in output (14).

TABLE 3 -- DOSE FROM NUCLEAR POWER PLANT EFFLUENTS IN THE YEAR 2000 (15)

	Area 10^3 sq. miles	Population 10^6	People per sq. mile	sq. miles per plant	rem/yr 10^6	mrem/yr/ capita
World	50.9	6222	122	38,000	2.04	0.33
USA	2.977	300	100	9,000	0.42	1.4
Europe	1.85	527	285	5,550	1.19	2.3
USSR	8.6	360	42	25,800	0.18	0.5
Rest of World	37.45	5035	134	113,000	0.56	0.1

In addition to exposures from the direct operations of the plants themselves, a larger dose contribution is derived from fuel processing plants. Waste management practices and the associated economics determine the amount of wastes ultimately released in this operation. Reasonable assumptions lead Parker to estimate per capita exposures from fuel reprocessing at .02 mrems/year (15) to the surface of the skin. Cowser et al. had previously estimated the world wide skin dose due to ^{85}Kr in the year 2000 as 1.8 mrem/year and due to tritium at 2 x 10^{-3} mrem/year (16).

OCCUPATIONAL EXPOSURES TO INTERNAL EMITTERS

A published 10-year summary of the exposures received by employees in the Atomic Energy Commission contractors facilities (1957-1966) documents 532 exposures in excess of 25% of the permissible annual dose commitment during that 10-year interval (17). Enriched uranium contamination accounted for almost half of these exposures followed by plutonium and tritium. These three were the agents involved in 92% of the cases, followed by polonium and iodine, and lastly 2 cases were recorded which involved ^{90}Sr. Iodine and polonium exposures when they occurred tended to be higher in amount than exposures to the other agents. The major facilities or operations in which these exposures occurred were production (64%), followed by research (14%) and maintenance (9%). The major route was inhalation (64%) followed by wounds (21%). It should be noted that no overexposures at this date have occurred at commercial nuclear power plants.

The facilities at which these exposures were recorded have carefully established health physics practices designed to minimize the chance of exposure and to maximize the probability of detecting exposures when they occur. The magnitude of occupational exposure in other industrial and medical installations is difficult to estimate since no single agency is responsible for collating these data.

Since 1950, the Occupational Health program of the U. S. Public Health Service has conducted continuing surveys of uranium miners in the Colorado Plateau region of the United States (18). The number of miners exposed in each year, and in different estimated exposure groups, has been tabulated and reported in great detail (19). Since the miners are exposed to increased levels of radon along with multiplicity of other noxious materials, it is not possible to estimate the magnitude of the hazard from each source with certainty. Thus, continued efforts have been made to reduce the composite of inhalation exposures to as low a level as is technically feasible, to minimize the well established risk of lung cancer in these workers.

MEDICAL ADMINISTRATIONS OF RADIOACTIVE COMPOUNDS

The growth of nuclear medicine and the administration of radioisotopes to people for diagnostic and therapeutic purposes has been very rapid over the past few years. The doubling time of X-ray procedures per capita is approximately 13 years, whereas it is close to 4 years for nuclear medicine procedures. Unfortunately, accurate current data regarding isotope utilization in patient studies are not readily available for nuclear medicine.

The results of a survey made in the United Kingdom in 1957 indicated that the GSD from the clinical use of radioisotopes was 0.18 mrem/year (20). At the time, the number of different clinical radioisotopic procedures was considerably less than today and reflected mainly the radiation dose from ^{131}I and ^{32}P. Surveys conducted in the United States in 1959 and 1966 indicate a four-fold increase in numbers of doses of radiopharmaceuticals to humans during that time period, not counting teletherapy and brachytherapy (21). Between 1966 and the present, the utilization of radiotracers in our clinic has grown rapidly and has doubled in this last 5 years. This is typical of current growth patterns in nuclear medicine in the U. S. A. Thus, an approximately 8 or 10 fold increase in utilization of radioisotopes in clinical nuclear medicine since 1959 may have occurred.

The predicted dosage to an average person living in the U. S. A. in the year 2000 is summarized in Table 4. All of the man-made sources, summed together will contribute less than 4% of the dose received from natural background. This can be looked upon as a small admixture to the hazards of life or

TABLE 4 -- ESTIMATED ANNUAL GENETICALLY SIGNIFICANT DOSE (GSD)
FROM RADIOACTIVE ISOTOPES (14)
U.S.A., YEAR 2000

Activity	mrem/yr/capita
Natural Background	
External *	97
Internal	22
Nuclear Power	0.6
Fuel Reprocessing	2
Diagnostic Use of Isotopes	1.8
Others	Negligible

* Including cosmic radiations

TABLE 5 -- CHANCE OF SERIOUS INJURY OR DEATH-PER YEAR (12)

Auto accident (disability)	1	chance in	100
Cancer, all types and causes	1	" "	700
Auto death	1	" "	4,000
Fire death	1	" "	25,000
The "Pill", death	1	" "	25,000
Drowning	1	" "	30,000
Electrocution	1	" "	200,000
Reactor Emanations; site boundary (5 to 10 mrem/yr.)	Less than 1	" "	1,000,000
Average for population within 50 miles of reactor	Less than 1	" "	10,000,000

can be viewed with alarm depending on the perspective
in which these estimates are viewed. The chance of
serious injury or death-per-year from different
causes is shown in Table 5 (12). The risk data are
relatively well established for each of these
categories, and the level of risk from radiations is
significantly less than from other accepted hazards
of modern life.

LATE EFFECTS OF RADIATION FROM RADIOACTIVE
ISOTOPES AND RELATION TO BODY STORES

The biologic consequences of radioactive
substances that are inhaled, ingested, or injected

differ from those of external irradiation. The distribution of internal emitters at the organ, cellular, and subcellular levels is highly variable, depending upon the biochemistry of the compound and the physiologic state of the system. For a given total dose, the dose rate is lower, and the duration of exposure is usually longer since it is determined by the effective half-life of the radioactive compound. A recent review by Nelson is an excellent summary of dose effect relationships observed in man and experimental animals following exposures to the radioactive isotopes of greatest current interest (22). The evidence that high doses of β and γ-emitting radionuclides can cause serious acute injuries ending in death is incontrovertable. Carcinogenesis is well established in man and animals following high radiation doses and the lesions so induced can not be distinguished from spontaneously arising tumors. Life shortening is seen following lower doses and is associated with a complex picture of morphologic and functional changes. An enormous amount of information has been collected concerning late effects of ionizing radiations from internal emitters. Most of the data are derived from experiments involving single radionuclides. Future studies involving combinations of radionuclides will be necessary to assess the extent to which co-factor interactions cause an amplified effect as has been seen with other combinations of injurious agents in man and animals.

For many years it has been known that workers who mined radioactive ores have an increased incidence of lung cancer. In the European mines in Schneeburg in Germany, and Joachimstal in Czechoslovakia, miners were exposed to high levels of radon and radon daughters, along with ore dust containing uranium, arsenic, nickel, silica, and other metals. A clear cut increase in lung cancer in the Schneeburg miners was noted as early as 1879, which preceded widespread cigarette smoking or use of diesel fuels as a power source in the mines (23). Similar lung cancer experiences have been reported for uranium miners in other countries including the U. S. A. (24). Unfortunately, data on exposure levels are uncertain or unavailable in most circumstances, and it is not possible to determine how much of the risk is due to which of the many noxious agents to which the miners are exposed. In the miners in the Colorado Plateau, careful studies have revealed an increased incidence of lung cancer, which the authors relate to exposure to radon and to cigarette smoking (25). They suggest that these two factors together cause an incidence of lung cancer which is higher than could be predicted from the arithmetic sum of the hazard from each agent. Because of the small number of non smokers in their sample, this suggestive finding could not be statistically substantiated.

To summarize current knowledge concerning the late effects of a single radioactive isotope, and to show the importance of body stores in mediation of radiobiologic effects, we shall consider the late effects of radioactive iodine ([131] I). Some of the reasons we base our discussions on this substance relate to the following facts: Iodine-131 is one of the agents produced in greatest amount in nuclear fission and is the radioactive isotope used most commonly in medicine; it is relatively long-lived (8-day half-life); it is incorporated into the food chain, and is absorbed rapidly and efficiently from the intestinal tract and localized with a high degree of selectivity in the thyroid gland. The degree of iodine uptake in the thyroid gland depends on body stores. If a person is iodine deficient, there is a very high probability that the iodine will be sequestered by the thyroid gland and incorporated into thyroid hormone. If body stores are saturated, lower amounts of radioactive iodine will be collected in the thyroid, and the dose to that gland will be reduced relative to the iodine deficient gland.

The sensitivity of the gland to the effects of the radioactive emissions also depends on the level of iodine content. Ordinarily, the thyroid is considered highly resistant to damage from ionizing radiation. This is based upon an inability to demonstrate changes in structure or function after moderate to high doses of [131] I (26). Maximum sensitivity of the gland is seen when an acute hyperplastic stimulation, as with chemical goitrogens, is received along with radiation exposure (27). Similarly, the more rapidly growing thyroid of the young animal appears to be more sensitive than the adult to cancer induction. Whether this is due to an inherent difference in the thyroid gland or to the amplification of induced defects by the more rapidly growing gland is not known.

Benign nodules have been noted in a large fraction of children who received mCi amounts of ^{131}I for treatment of hyperthyroidism (28). These children did not receive thyroid supplementation following therapy and hence may have had increased TSH levels and associated hyperplasia. Children treated with similar radioactive doses with thyroid supplementation showed no evidence of adenoma development in a comparable study group (29). The evidence for co-factor interactions increasing the induction of adenomas in man seems fairly well established.

Until recently it was generally accepted that the incidence of thyroid cancer was higher in endemic goiter regions (30). This was presumed to be related to the higher level of TSH stimulation, although other factors might also play a role in determining which individuals developed malignancies. Subsequent studies have not revealed this same geographical pattern, and Doniach, in reviewing the evidence pro and con, concludes that the effect, if present, is not prominent. However, the incidence of follicular cancer of the thyroid may have fallen since the introduction of iodized food products (31), while the incidence of papillary cancer has risen. The latter is presumed to be due to a change in the pathologic criteria currently in vogue, and if dietary iodine deficiency leads to thyroid cancer, the tumor type is likely to be follicular.

The radiation dose to the thyroid from ^{131}I therapy is more than ten times greater than the radiation dose from external X-ray treatment in those cases where thyroid cancer has been reported as a possible sequelae (32,33). The radiobiologic basis for the lower hazard factor from ^{131}I is not understood. The results of the medical survey of the people of Rongelap and Utirik Islands 11 and 12 years after exposure to fallout radiation revealed a higher than expected incidence of thyroid tumors in persons exposed as children to mixed exposures, i.e. iodine radioisotopes and external gamma radiations (34). Whether this markedly elevated incidence is due to

177

underestimation of the radiation dose, summation of the effects of internal and external exposures, or related to the interplay of other major factors is not known.

Similarly, studies in the A-bomb survivors in Hiroshima and Nagasaki have shown an increased thyroid cancer incidence, although the magnitude of the effect is much smaller (35). Although the number of cases was small, the thyroid cancer incidence was highest in those receiving the largest exposures, and these patients were younger on the average than the more distantly exposed thyroid cancer patients. An intriguing correlation that came to light in the leukemia surveys was that 4 patients had both leukemia and thyroid cancer. These 4 patients received large exposures and represent 25% or more of the thyroid cancer diagnoses in the heavily exposed survivors. The basis for this unusual combination of diseases is unknown, and is sufficiently intriguing to invite careful investigation.

Leukemia, itself, can be induced by ^{131}I exposure. Patients with long-standing, untreated thyrotoxicosis have been reported to have an increased incidence of lymphoma (36). Patients with thyrotoxicosis itself have a higher than normal incidence of leukemia, which does not appear to be correlated with whether or not they receive ^{131}I in therapy in the usual dose range (37). However, the larger doses used in therapy of thyroid cancer lead to a marked increase in leukemia incidence, and there can be no question but that ^{131}I can cause leukemia if the dose is sufficiently high (38).

Thus, it is clear that high doses of a single radioactive isotope can cause an adverse effect. The hazard at lower exposures can be enhanced by synergy with other common or unusual co-factors. Radiation sensitivity is often enhanced when the biological system is growing rapidly, as in young children or even more so in the fetus. With radioactive isotopes, metabolic factors lead to non-uniform dose distributions which make it extra difficult to establish meaningful dose-effect relationships. Based upon biological experience, a possible carcinogenic hazard from ^{131}I has been reported following administrations of 1-5 mCi (33). These correspond to thyroid doses on the order of 1,000 to

10,000 rads. Doses in excess of 1,000 rad are now known to induce hypothyroidism, but at lower doses we have not been able to detect significant biological damage from ^{131}I. Of all the man-made radioactive materials, ^{131}I has received the greatest attention. It is estimated that population exposure to this agent in the year 2000 is likely to be less than .001 rad/capita, which is a factor of 1 million less than doses which may cause hypothyroidism or thyroid cancer.

REFERENCES

1. United Nations. (1958). Report of the United Nations Scientific Committee on the Effects of Atomic Radiation. General Assembly, Thirteenth Session, Suppl. No. 17 (A/3838).

2. United Nations. (1962). Report of the United Nations Scientific Committee on the Effects of Atomic Radiation. General Assembly, Seventeenth Session, Suppl. No. 16 (A/5216).

3. United Nations. (1964). Report of the United Nations Scientific Committee on the Effects of Atomic Radiation. General Assembly, Nineteenth Session, Suppl. No. 14 (A/5814).

4. United Nations. (1966). Report of the United Nations Scientific Committee on the Effects of Atomic Radiation. General Assembly, Twenty-first Session, Suppl. No. 14 (A/6314).

5. United Nations. (1969). Report of the United Nations Scientific Committee on the Effects of Atomic Radiation. General Assembly, Twenty-fourth Session, Suppl. No. 13 (A/7613).

6. Morgan, K. A. and Turner, J. E. (1967). Principles of Radiation Protection. John Wiley and Sons, New York.

7. Spier, F. W. (1968). Radioisotopes in the Human Body. Academic Press, New York.

8. Ellis, R. E. (1965). An appraisal of the current fall out levels and the biological significance. Phys. Med. Biol. 10: 153.

9. U. S. Atomic Energy Commission. (1969). Forecast of Growth of Nuclear Power. Washington, 1139.

10. Seaborg, Glenn. (1969). Testimony. Environmental Effects of Producing Electric Power, Hearings Before the Joint Committee on Atomic Energy, Congress of the United States, Washington, D. C., 86.

11. Atomic Energy Comission. (1971). AEC proposes numerical guidance to keep radioactivity in light water-cooled nuclear power reactor effluents as low as practicable. News Release 0-87. June 7.

12. Bond, V. (1971). Health Physics Society Newsletter, February.

13. Rogers, L. and Gamertsfelder, C. (1970). U. S. Regulations for the Control of Radioactivity to the Environment in Effluents from Nuclear Facilities. IAEA Symposium, U. N. Headquarters, New York, 10.

14. Parker, F. L. (1971). Public health implications of radioactive waste releases, IVth Geneva Conference on Peaceful Uses of Atomic Energy.

15. Straub, C. P. (1970). Public health implications of radioactive waste releases.

16. Cowser, K. E., Boegly, W. J. and Jacobs, D. G. (1966). Annual Progress Report for Period Ending July 31, 1966. U. S. Atomic Energy Commission, ORNL. 4007.

17. Ross, D. A. (1967). A statistical summary of U. S. Atomic Energy Commission contractors' internal exposures experience. 1957-1966. In: Excerpta Medica Foundation, (ed.), Diagnosis and Treatment of Deposited Radionuclides. Proc. Symp. Richland, Washington, May 15-17, 1967.

18. Holaday, D. A. (1969). History of the exposure of miners to radon. Health Phys. 16: 547.

19. Joint Committee on Atomic Energy, Sub-Committee on Research, Development, and Radiation. (1967). Hearings on Radiation Hazards in Uranium Mines, May and June 1967. U. S. Govt. Print. Off., Washington, D. C.

20. Ministry of Health, Department of Health for Scotland. (1960). Radiological Hazards to Patients. Her Majesty's Stationery Office, London.

21. U. S. Dept. of Health, Education, and Welfare, PHS. (1970). Survey of the Use of Radionuclides in Medicine. BRH/DMRE 70-1. Rockville, Maryland.

22. Nelson, A. (1970). Late effects of radiation from internal gamma and beta ray emitters. In: R. J. M. Fry et al. (eds.), Late Effects of Radiation. Taylor and Francis, Ltd., London.

23. Hueper, W. C. (1942). Occupational Tumors and Related Diseases. C. C. Thomas, Springfield, Illinois.

24. Donaldson, A. W. (1969). The epidemiology of lung cancer among uranium miners. Health Phys. 16: 563.

25. Lundin, F. E. et al. (1969). Mortality of uranium miners in relation to radiation exposure, hard-rock mining, and cigarette smoking -- 1950 through September 1967. Health Phys. 16: 571.

26. Rubin, P. and Casarett, G. (1968). Clinical Radiation Pathology. W. B. Saunders, Philadelphia.

27. Doniach, I. (1968). Damaging effect of X-irradiation of less than 1000 rads on goitrogenic capacity of rat thyroid gland. In: S. Young and D. R. Inman, (eds.), Thyroid Neoplasia. Academic Press, London.

28. Sheline, G. E. et al. (1962). Thyroid nodules occurring late after treatment of thyrotoxicosis with radioiodine. J. Clin. Endocrinol. Metab. 22: 8.

29. Starr, P., Jaffe, H. L. and Oettinger, L. (1964). Late results of I-131 treatment of hyperthyroidism in 73 children and adolescents. J. Nuc. Med. 5: 81.

30. Wynder, E. L. (1952). Medical progress. Some practical aspects of cancer prevention. New Eng. J. Med. 246: 576.

31. Doniach, I. (1970). Aetiological consideration of thyroid cancer. In: D. Smithers, (ed.), Monographs on Neoplastic Disease. E. and S. Livingstone, Edinburgh and London, VI.

32. Pifer, J. W. and Hemplemann, L. H. (1964). Radiation-induced thyroid carcinoma. Ann. N. Y. Acad. Sci. 114: 838.

33. Lima, J. B., Catz, B. and Perzik, S. L. (1970). Thyroid cancer following ^{131}I therapy of hyperthyroidism. J. Nuc. Med. 11: 46.

34. Conard, R. A., Rall, J. E. and Sutow, W. W. (1966). Thyroid nodules as a late sequela of radioactive fallout. New Eng. J. Med. 274: 1391.

35. Socolow, E. L. et al. (1963). Thyroid carcinoma in man after exposure to ionizing radiation. New Eng. J. Med. 268: 406.

36. Ultmann, J. E., Hyman, G. A. and Calder, B. (1963). The occurrence of lymphoma in patients with longstanding hyperthyroidism. Blood 21: 282.

37. Saenger, E. L., Thomas, G. E. and Tompkins, E. A. (1968). Incidence of leukemia following treatment of hyperthyroidism: Preliminary report of the cooperative thyrotoxicosis therapy follow-up study. J. Amer. Med. Assoc. 205: 855.

38. Pochin, E. E. (1961). The occurrence of
     leukemia following radioiodine therapy. In: R.
     P. H. Rivers, (ed.), Advances in Thyroid
     Research, Transactions of the Fourth
     International Goiter Conference. Pergamon
     Press, London, 392.

CHAPTER 12. STORAGE AS A FACTOR IN DISEASE DUE TO MINERAL DUSTS

J. C. MCDONALD, G. W. GIBBS, J. MANFREDA, and
F. M. M. WHITE, Department of Epidemiology and
Health, McGill University, Montreal, Canada

Diseases caused by dust and fibres tend to be chronic and progressive and to occur after long and substantial exposure. Various kinds of disease mechanisms are compatible with this pattern. The process once initiated might sustain itself; immediate or delayed effects of exposure might accumulate; storage of dust or derivatives within the body, with continuous or periodic release, might maintain pathogenesis. As these are not mutually exclusive hypotheses and probably all three contribute to some extent, their separate assessment is a formidable task. Effects attributable to stored dust could probably be detected with confidence only in subjects removed for some time from exposure, and it would still be necessary to exclude the possibility of a self-sustaining process.

Since we are concerned with detailed analysis of dose-response relationships, epidemiological studies of considerable quality and sophistication are needed. Few have been attempted, no doubt because more basic questions of cause and effect have yet to be answered. Unless the causal agents in a disease have been rather well defined it is almost impossible to consider them quantitatively.

Tempting though it may be to dismiss the storage issue as a refinement of purely academic interest, even basic etiological studies cannot ignore it. It is usually implicit that any effect due to storage of the agent is proportional to indices of total intake. If this assumption is correct, sufficient understanding of dose-response can probably be obtained for control purposes, without taking storage into account. If it is seriously incorrect, there would be difficulty in defining a safe level and even the existence of a causal relationship put in doubt.

As the problem is complex, we have limited this review to mineral dusts and fibrous silicates as they relate to pulmonary fibrosis, and asbestos as a factor in lung cancer and malignant pleural mesothelioma. We have had to lean more heavily than we would have wished on morphological and pathological evidence, though recognizing that this can be misleading, even in situations where cause and effect are well established.

STORAGE PROCESS

Retention in the nose is almost complete for particles more than about 10 μm in diameter (1,2) though fibres within this size may pass even if 10-20 times longer (3). Deposition in the respiratory tract and alveoli then depends on settlement, impact, interception, and diffusion (4). Spherical particles, too small to be affected by inertia but too large (above 0.5 μm) to be affected by molecular bombardment, fall out at a rate determined by radius, shape, and density. The falling speed of fibres is determined by their diameter, and curly fibres are more liable to interception in the branching respiratory passages than straight fibres. For those reasons fine curly fibres, such as chrysotile as presently milled, are probably less likely to penetrate deeply into the lung than the straighter and wider fibres of amosite and some forms of crocidolite (5,6). Concentration of particles and electric charge, and growth of hygroscopic particles due to humidity, all of which affect aggregation, may influence the rate of deposition (2). Ambient conditions of temperature and humidity, extreme in some mining environments, will have similar effects. There remain the considerable but less well defined factors of human variation, partly due to physiological and anatomic differences, partly to breathing and smoking habits, and partly to physical effort.

186

Most particles deposited in the alveoli are rapidly phagocytosed by cells of the alveolar walls. These become detached and migrate upwards in the tracheobronchial tract. Depending on the cytotoxicity of the ingested particles and the availability of phagocytic cells, migration of these particles may be intracellular, or extracellular (7-10). Proximal movement of dust-cells and extracellular particles is facilitated by the flow of surfactant secreted by other alveolar cells (11-13). Although active amoeboid movement may occur initially, it is likely that dust-cells lose this capacity after ingestion of sufficient particulate matter.

Though most dust-cells, debris, and extracellular particles are thus transported to the distal end of the mucociliary membrane of the terminal bronchioles and eliminated from the lung, a small proportion gain entry to the interstitium (14). Some particles appear to penetrate the alveolar or bronchiolar walls and some enter at the junction of the alveolar ducts and respiratory bronchioles (15). The route by which dust-cells enter is less clear, although evidence tends to favour the non-epithelialized connective tissue junctions between the alveolar ducts and respiratory bronchioles (13). Whether interstitial entry of dust-cells is confined to those of histiocytic origin, thus excluding the vast majority which originate from alveolar epithelium, is debatable. Silica particles may penetrate the interstitium in an extracellular manner, but it is evident that in the case of asbestos fibres dust-cells play a major role (14,16). Aside from active amoeboid movement, this migration is assisted by centrifugal flow of tissue fluid and by fluctuations in intrapulmonary pressure with respiration. Where alveoli lie against perivascular and peribronchiolar sheaths, dust-cells may penetrate directly into the connective tissue without entering the lumen. Interstitial sequestration, regardless of mechanism, accounts for only a small proportion of the total alveolar clearance but this is the proportion destined for long-term storage in the lungs or regional nodes.

SILICOSIS AND ANTHRACOSIS

PATHOLOGY -- Storage of silica and coal dust is associated with focal lesions in the peribronchiolar and perivascular connective tissue, subpleural spaces and tracheo-bronchial nodes. This distribution is probably due to fluctuating intrapulmonary pressure, diminished clearance capacity of alveoli adjacent to semi-rigid structures, and to distal lymphatic obstruction by dust-cells and fibrosis (17,18). Interference with normal drainage toward the hilar nodes leads to accumulation of particles and metabolic products and results in further fibrosis and increased lung weight (19). The silicotic nodule has an acellular hyalinized centre surrounded by a zone of cellular fibrous tissue and an external zone of irregular connective tissue (20). Movement of silica particles to the periphery, possibly in phagocytes, explains their absence centrally and the progressive enlargement of the nodule. Several mechanisms of fibrogenesis have been postulated; the two currently most widely held depend either on surface activity of silica or on the production from it of silicic acid. Cellular damage from either of these may lead on to autoimmune reactions.

The basic lesion of coal-workers simple pneumoconiosis is the coal macule, evolved by incorporation of dust-filled macrophages into the wall of respiratory bronchioles and adjacent alveoli with consequent fibrosis (21,22). Fibrosis is less dense than in silicotic nodules, and may consist only of loose reticulin and collagen, when present, is rarely of concentric appearance. Invested bronchioles may undergo dilatation which results in focal emphysema and the characteristic honeycombed appearance (23). Whether the process is primarily due to the silica content of coal dust or purely to dust accumulation with attendant structural and functional changes is not resolved. Both coal-workers' simple pneumoconiosis and silicosis may proceed to massive fibrotic forms. The genesis of such conditions is beyond the scope of this discussion, but may involve tuberculosis, vascular occlusion, mixed dust exposure, and immunological phenomena, in addition to the underlying storage of dust and fibrotic reaction to it.*

EPIDEMIOLOGY -- Rivers et al. (24) provided the first quantitative evidence of how radiological and pathological features were related to both total amount and mineral composition of dust in the lungs of coal-workers with simple pneumoconiosis. Nagelschmidt (25) found that the amount of quartz in cases of silicosis increased from 3 g to 6 g with severity of fibrosis. In coal-workers, some twenty times as much dust was present and again quantity and severity were related. In a small series of cases of pneumoconiosis associated with quartz-free dust, Nagelschmidt found an average dust content of 20% of dried lung weight, but there were too few cases to assess the relationship to severity. It was shown by Klosterkotter and Einbrodt (26) that quartz increased the penetration and retention of inert dusts, probably because of its cytotoxic effect on alveolar macrophages. Neutralization of this cytotoxicity with polyvinyl-pyridine-N-oxide (PVNO) results in decreased dust retention. The work of Rivers et al. was extended in 1965 by Rossiter et al. (27), who made a large survey of lungs from a wide range of British coalfields. Coal, iron, and mineral content were all related to radiological category. The best correlation was with iron content, probably of endogenous origin; the next best was the mineral content, of which an average of 54%, was silica. More recently the same workers concluded that the iron probably reflected only the presence of coal and mineral dust (28).

ASBESTOSIS AND TALCOSIS

PATHOLOGY -- Pulmonary fibrosis due to asbestos (29) and talc (30) tends to follow a diffuse interstitial pattern often accompanied by fibrotic pleural thickening (31,32). Fine fibrosis develops round the respiratory bronchioles, alveolar ducts, and sacs, and extends outwards. Airways become dilated, resulting in a honeycombed appearance with some bronchiectasis. Fine nodulation may occur, particularly in the

---

* See also "Pulmonary Reactions to Coal Dust" in this Series. (Eds.)

lower parts of the lungs. Pleural and septal fibrosis are relatively late effects and massive fibrosis of the lungs may also ensue. In talcosis, the fibrosis is more nodular and large amounts of doubly-refractile dust with sparse talc bodies can usually be seen (23). This contrasts with asbestosis, where most of the fibres are coated to form asbestos bodies and doubly-refractile fibres are seldom present. Neither talc nor asbestos bodies can be readily distinguished from ferrunginous bodies caused by other mineral fibres and these may be present with or without pulmonary fibrosis (32,33). The terms "asbestos body" and "talc body" are, therefore, best reserved for circumstances where their origin is well supported by an occupational history or by appropriate physico-chemical analysis. Asbestos bodies are found most frequently in lungs but also in maxillary and frontal sinuses, tonsils, spleen, and peritoneum (32). Current evidence suggests that asbestos bodies develop intracellularly, even when formed around large fibres which require the action of several cells (34,35). Granules of hemosiderin and ferritin gather along the fibre, originating probably from broken-down erythrocytes, circulating transferrin, or other body stores (20). Protein is adsorbed onto the forming body and there may also be some collagen. Naked fibres appear to become innocuous after encapsulation within ferruginous bodies, but the bodies, may break down years later with release of the fibrogenic core (36).

EPIDEMIOLOGY -- There is a close relation between various indices of dust exposure in asbestos miners and millers and the incidence and severity of radiographic and functional manifestations of asbestosis (37-39). To what extent there is progression after removal from exposure has not been established. Analyses of dust and fibre in the lungs at autopsy have been rare in asbestosis. Beatie and Knox (40) found an average mineral content of 0.4% of dried lung weight, with no clear increase with severity of fibrosis, and a decrease in dust proportional to the period between the end of exposure and death. The hilum and pleura contained as much or more dust than the lungs. Nagelschmidt (41), in a study of lungs from twenty moderate or severe cases of asbestosis, found no more than traces of asbestos in half of them. There is considerable evidence, nevertheless, that asbestos bodies and fibres may remain in the tissues for many years, so that gradual fragmentation and dissolution might well continue the fibrotic process after removal from further exposure.

LUNG CANCER

The microscopic and macroscopic features of lung cancer in asbestos and talc workers does not differ from that in the general population (29,42). High death rates from lung cancer (9% to 25%) have been reported in known cases of asbestosis (43-46), and in some series the tumor was more frequent in lower than upper lobes (29,42,47). Selection of cases may have contributed to these associations which, if true, might be due either to common etiology or to predisposition of fibrosis to malignancy. Animal experiments have failed to throw much light so far on the carcinogenic potential of asbestos. Until recently it was not sufficiently appreciated that asbestos dust prepared for laboratory experiments had often been contaminated by oils during storage (48), and by metals such as nickel, chromium and cobalt (49), in the special milling process.

There is abundant evidence of an association between asbestos exposure in a variety of industrial occupations and increased frequency of lung cancer. Some notable studies were those of Doll (50) and Knox et al. (51) in British textile plants, Newhouse (52) in a British asbestos factory, Enterline and Kendrick (53) in various kinds of asbestos plants in the USA, Selikoff et al. (54) in American insulation workers, and McDonald et al. (55) in the Quebec mine and mills. The highest risk appeared to be in the insulation workers whose exposure though probably heavy was not quantitated. The studies of both Knox et al. and Newhouse showed that risk was related to high or long exposure and absent with short exposure or after environmental conditions had improved. In the Quebec survey, excess mortality from lung cancer was virtually confined to men who had worked an equivalent of forty years at an average dust level of fifty fibres per ml or more, assuming the fibre content of dust to be about 10%, i.e. ten times the Threshold Limit Value proposed by the American Conference of Governmental Industrial Hygienists in 1970. There is regrettably no comparable information for workers in crocidolite or amosite mines and mills. In the large study of insulation workers by Selikoff et al. (56), the considerable excess of lung cancer was confined to the smoking segment of the population. If this were to prove generally true, it would imply that asbestos was either a carrier of carcinogenic substances or a co-carcinogen.

No quantitative relationships have been established between asbestos fibres in the lung and the presence of lung cancer. Appropriate techniques have been developed by Langer (57), Gold (58,59) and Pooley et al. (60), and preliminary findings suggest that cases in asbestos workers have high fibre counts. However, it may prove difficult to show that this signifies anything more than past exposure. Though the point does not appear to have been specifically studied, cases of lung cancer have often developed in persons years after exposure to asbestos terminated. This evidence is difficult to interpret without objective methods of separating cases attributable to asbestos from the majority which are not.

MALIGNANT MESOTHELIOMA

Several adequately controlled retrospective inquiries have shown that a substantial proportion of persons with primary malignant mesothelioma tumours have worked with asbestos, or had less direct contact at home or in the neighbourhood of asbestos plants (61-64). The cohort of insulation workers studied by Selikoff et al. (65) suffered an extraordinarily high rate of these rare tumours, and the experience of London crocidolite factory workers studied by Newhouse and Wagner (66) was almost as bad. In contrast, few mesotheliomas have been diagnosed in the Quebec chrysotile industry and none at all in the chrysotile mines and mills of Russia (67), Northern Italy (68), or Cyprus (69). In Finland too, the tumours are very rare though anthophyllite is produced and calcified pleural plaques are common (70). Only in Canada (63) and Scotland (64) has any systematic attempt been made at total ascertainment, followed by investigation of possible exposure. In both countries the incidence was low -- about one per million population per annum -- but in Scotland there was rather more evidence of contact with asbestos. In all studies to date, most evidence of the association has been in the working environment and less often under domestic or neighbourhood conditions alone. This suggests that the risk may be dose-related. With few exceptions, time between first exposure and onset is very long, usually from 20-40 years, and in many cases time since last dust exposure is also long. Further evidence of association between stored asbestos fibre and malignant mesothelial tumours lies in the frequency with which ferruginous bodies have been observed in lungs from fatal cases, as compared with other causes of death (61,62,71-73). Recent investigations aimed at the identification and quantitation of asbestos fibres in tissue suggest that the number of fibres per unit of lung tissue may prove even higher in cases of peritoneal malignant mesothelioma than in asbestosis or lung cancer.

Until the etiology of malignant mesothelial tumours is better understood, the importance of stored fibre must remain speculative. An explanation is needed for the high incidence in persons exposed to asbestos under certain circumstances but not in others. It is possible that for physical reasons, it may be less likely for chrysotile to be retained in the respiratory tract than crocidolite and perhaps other amphiboles. Alternatively, some additional factor, present only in certain situations of asbestos exposure, may be the more essential carcinogen.

CONCLUSION

Pulmonary storage of dusts and fibres may produce a three-fold effect. Firstly, significant dust storage in the tracheo-bronchial nodes, with or without fibrosis, may contribute to proximal lymphatic stagnation and accumulation of metabolic products, dust-cells and dust with associated fibrotic effects. Secondly, in order to exert a pathologic effect, regardless of underlying mechanism, the dust or fibre concerned must reside at least temporarily within the confines of susceptible tissues. Thirdly, simple accumulation of relatively non-toxic and non-fibrogenic dusts, such as pure coal dust, may lead by virtue of sheer quantity and consequent imbalance of respiratory forces to structural and functional changes. With toxic and fibrogenic dusts, such as silica, their pathogenicity may limit the extent to which dust can accumulate before severe incapacity ensues. Individual susceptibility is still not understood and may depend on alveolar clearance rates, immunological variation, presence of pre-existing disease, microanatomical differences, and a host of other intrinsic and extrinsic factors.

The relation between dust or fibre storage in the lungs and the amount of fibrosis is complex. In coal-workers' simple pneumoconiosis, storage and fibrotic response appear directly related, but individual susceptibility prevents exact formulation of the relationship. The same may be true of silicosis and talcosis, though the relationships here are less precise. In asbestosis, the small amount of chrysotile fibre found at autopsy infers that dissolution has occurred, so that the existence of a fibrogenic breakdown product has been hypothesized to explain fibrosis in the face of so little remaining asbestos fibre. The ferruginous body associated with the pulmonary retention of asbestos, talc, and other fibres may therefore constitute a storage capacity of significance.

The extent to which stored fibre is responsible for the increased rate of respiratory cancers associated with asbestos and talc has practical implications for exposed workers and, perhaps, in the case of mesothelial tumours, for the general public. Despite ignorance of the precise role played by the various types of asbestos fibre in carcinogenesis, the fact remains that the tumours in question commonly occur many years after last recorded exposure and in lungs which often contain fibres or ferruginous bodies. Though the fibres may act only as a carrier of carcinogenic substances, their retention in the lung could still be important.

REFERENCES

1. Prattle, R. E. (1961). The retention of gases and particles in the human nose. In: C. N. Davies, (ed.), Inhaled Particles and Vapours, I. Pergamon, Oxford, 302.

2. Green, H. L. and Lane, W. R. (1964). Particulate clouds, dusts, smokes and mists. E. and F. N. Spon, London, 349.

3. Timbrell, V. (1965). The inhalation of fibrous dusts. Ann. N. Y. Acad. Sci. 132: 255.

4. Timbrell, V. (1970). The inhalation of fibres. In: H. A. Shapiro, (ed.), Proc. Int. Conf. Pneumoniosis, Johannesburg, 1969. Oxford University Press, Cape Town, 3.

5. Wagner, J. C. and Skidmore, J. W. (1965). Asbestos dust deposition and retention in rats. Ann. N. Y. Acad. Sci. 132: 77.

6. Davies, C. N. (1970). Tissue responses to asbestos. (A report of a meeting). Ann. Occup. Hyg. 13: 241.

7. Policard, A. (1952). The mechanism of dispersion of coal particles in the lungs of miners. Brit. J. Indust. Med. 9: 108.

8. Labelle, C. W. and Brieger, H. (1960). The fate of inhaled particles in the early post-exposure period. Arch. Env. Health 1: 423.

9. Mottura, G. (1952). Penetration of dust particles and sites of dust stores in pneumoconiosis. Brit. J. Indust. Med. 9: 65.

10. Heppleston, A. G. (1963). The disposal of inhaled particulate matter; a unifying hypothesis. Amer. J. Path. 42: 119.

11. Mendenhall, R. M. (1963). Pulmonary mechanics: Some physical and biochemical factors. Arch. Env. Health 6: 74.

12. Macklin, C. C. (1955). Lung fluid, alveolar dust drift, and initial lesions in the lungs. Canad. Med. Assoc. J. 72: 664.

13. Macklin, C. C. (1955). Pulmonary sumps, dust accumulations, alveolar fluid, and lymph vessels. Acta. Anat. 23: 1.

14. Gross, P. and Westrick, M. (1954). The permeability of lung parenchyma to particulate matter. Amer. J. Pathol. 2: 195.

15. Holt, P. F., Mills, J. and Young, D. K. (1964). The early effects of chrysotile asbestos dust on the rat lung. J. Pathol. Bacteriol. 87: 15.

16. Davies, J. M. G. (1963). An electron microscope study of the effect of asbestos dust on the lung. Brit. J. Exp. Pathol. 44: 454.

17. Gross, P., Westrick, M. L. and McNerney, J. M. (1958). Experimental silicosis: The morphogenesis of the silicotic nodule. Amer. Med. Assoc. Arch. Indust. Health 18: 374.

18. King, E. J. et al. (1958). The tissue reaction in the lungs of rats after the inhalation of coal dust containing 2% of quartz. Brit. J. Indust. Med. 15: 172.

19. Schepers, G. W. H. (1960). Theories of the causes of silicosis -- Part II. Indust. Med. and Surg. 29: 259.

20. Gough, J. and Heppleston, A. G. (1960). The pathology of the pneumoconioses. In: E. J. King and C. M. Fletcher, (eds.), Industrial Pulmonary Diseases -- A Symposium. Churchill, London.

21. Heppleston, A. G. (1951). Coalworkers' pneumoconiosis -- Pathological and etiological considerations. Arch. Indust. Hyg. 4: 270.

22. Liebow, A. A. (1970). Pathology of coalworkers pneumoconiosis. Indust. Med. and Surg. 39: 118.

23. Gough, J. (1947). Pneumoconiosis in coalworkers in Wales. Occup. Med. 4: 86.

24. Rivers, D. et al. (1960). Dust content, radiology, and pathology in simple pneumoconiosis of coal workers. Brit. J. Indust. Med. 17: 87.

25. Nagelschmidt, G. (1960). The relation between lung dust and lung pathology in pneumoconiosis. Brit. J. Indust. Med. 17: 247.

26. Klosterkotter, W. and Einbrodt, H. J. (1965). Retention, penetration, and elimination of inhaled dusts. In: C. N. Davies, (ed.), Inhaled Particles and Vapours, II. Pergamon, Oxford, 215.

27. Rossiter, C. E. et al. (1965). Dust content, radiology, and pathology in simple pneumoconiosis of coal workers. In: C. N. Davies, (ed.), Inhaled Particles and Vapours, II. Pergamon, Oxford, 419.

28. Casswell, G., Bergman, I. and Rossiter, C. E. (1971). The relation of radiological appearance in simple pneumoconiosis of coal-workers to the content and composition of the lungs. In: W. H. Walton, (ed.), Inhaled Particles, Unwin, Old Woking, 713.

29. Hourihane, D. O'B. and McCaughey, W. T. E. (1966). Pathological aspects of asbestosis. Postgrad. Med. J. 42: 613.

30. Kleinfeld, M. et al. (1964). Lung function in talc workers. Arch. Env. Health 9: 559.

31. Gough, J. (1965). Differential diagnosis in the pathology of asbestosis. Ann. N. Y. Acad. Sci. 132: 368.

32. Meurman, L. (1966). Asbestos bodies and pleural plaques in a Finnish series of autopsy cases. Acta Pathol. Microbiol. Scand. Suppl. 181: 1.

33. Gross, P., Cralley, L. J. and de Treville, R. T. P. (1967). "Asbestos" bodies: Their

non-specificity. Amer. Indust. Hyg. Assoc. J. 28: 541.

34. Davis, J. M. G. (1964). The ultrastructure of asbestos bodies from guinea pig lungs. Brit. J. Exp. Pathol. 45: 634.

35. Suzuki, Y. and Churg, J. (1969). Structure and development of the asbestos body. Amer. J. Pathol. 55: 79.

36. Knox, J. F. and Beattie, J. (1954). Distribution of mineral particles and fibers in lung after exposure to asbestos dust. Arch. Indust. Hyg. 10: 30.

37. McDonald, J. C. et al. (1972). Respiratory symptoms in chrysotile asbestos mine and mill workers of Quebec. Arch. Env. Health 24: 358.

38. Becklake, M. R. et al. (1972). Lung function in chrysotile asbestos mine and mill workers of Quebec. Arch. Env. Health 24: 401.

39. Rossiter, C. E. et al. (1972). Radiographic changes in chrysotile asbestos mine and mill workers of Quebec. Arch. Env. Health 24: 388.

40. Beattie, J. and Knox, I. F. (1961). Studies of mineral content and particle size distribution in the lungs of asbestos textile workers. In: C. N. Davies, (ed.), Inhaled Particles and Vapours, I. Pergamon, Oxford, 419.

41. Nagelschmidt, G. (1965). Some observations of the dust content and composition in lungs with asbestosis, made during work on coal miners pneumoconiosis. Ann. N. Y. Acad. Sci. 132: 64.

42. O'Donnell, W. M., Mann, R. H. and Grosh, J. L. (1966). An extrinsic factor in the pathogenesis of bronchogenic carcinoma and mesothelioma. Cancer 19: 1143.

43. Merewether, E. R. A. (1949). Asbestosis and Carcinoma of the Lung. Annual Report for the Chief Inspector of Factories for the Year 1947, London, HMSO, 79.

44. Gloyne, S. R. (1951). Pneumoconiosis: Histological survey of necropsy material. Lancet 1: 811.

45. Buchanan, W. D. (1965). Asbestos and primary intrathoracic neoplasms. Ann. N. Y. Acad. Sci. 132: 507.

46. Vigliani, E. C., Mottura, G. and Maranzana, P. (1965). Association of pulmonary tumours with asbestosis in Piedmont and Lombardy. Ann. N. Y. Acad. Sci. 132: 558.

47. Jacob, G. and Anspach, M. (1965). Pulmonary neoplasia among Dresden asbestos workers. Ann. N. Y. Acad. Sci. 132: 536.

48. Gibbs, G. W. (1964). Some problems associated with the storage of asbestos in polyethylene bags. Amer. Indust. Hyg. Assoc. J. 30: 458.

49. Cralley, L. J., Keenan, R. G. and Lynch, J. R. (1967). Exposure to metals in the manufacture of asbestos textile products. Amer. Indust. Hyg. Assoc. J. 28: 452.

50. Doll, R. (1955). Mortality from lung cancer in asbestos workers. Brit. J. Indust. Med. 12: 81.

51. Knox, J. F. et al. (1968). Mortality from lung cancer and other causes among workers in an asbestos textile factory. Brit. J. Indust. Med. 25: 293.

52. Newhouse, M. L. (1969). A study of the mortality of workers in an asbestos factory. Brit. J. Indust. Med. 26: 294.

53. Enterline, P. E. and Kendrick, M. A. (1967). Asbestos dust exposures at various levels and mortality. Arch. Env. Health 15: 181.

54. Selikoff, I. J., Churg, J. and Hammond, E. C. (1964). Asbestos exposure and neoplasia. J. Amer. Med. Assoc. 188: 22.

55. McDonald, J. C. et al. (1971). Mortality in the chrysotile asbestos mines and mills of Quebec. Arch. Env. Health 22: 677.

56. Selikoff, I. J., Hammond, E. C. and Churg, J. (1968). Asbestos exposure, smoking, and neoplasia. J. Amer. Med. Assoc. 204: 106.

57. Langer, A. M., Rubin, I. and Selikoff, I. J. (1970). Electron microprobe analysis of asbestos bodies. In: H. A. Shapiro, (ed.), Proc. Int. Conf. Pneumoconiosis, Johannesburg, 1969. Oxford University Press, Cape Town, 57.

58. Gold, C. (1968). The quantitation of asbestos in tissue. J. Clin. Pathol. 21: 537.

59. Gold, C. (1969). Asbestos levels in human lungs. J. Clin. Pathol. 22: 507.

60. Pooley, F. D. et al. (1970). The detection of asbestos in tissues. In: H. A. Shapiro, (ed.), Proc. Int. Conf. Pneumoconiosis, Johannesburg, 1969. Oxford University Press, Cape Town, 108.

61. Elmes, P. C., McCaughey, W. T. E. and Wade, O. L. (1965). Diffuse mesothelioma of the pleura and asbestos. Brit. Med. J. 1: 350.

62. Newhouse, M. L. and Thompson, H. (1965). Mesothelioma of pleura and peritonium following exposure to asbestos in the London area. Brit. J. Indust. Med. 22: 261.

63. McDonald, A. D. et al. (1970). Epidemiology of primary malignant mesothelial tumours in Canada. Cancer 26: 914.

64. McEwen, J. et al. (1970). Mesothelioma in Scotland. Brit. Med. J. 4: 575.

65. Selikoff, I. J., Hammond, E. C. and Churg, J. (1970). Mortality experiences of asbestos insulation workers, 1943-1968. In: H. A. Shapiro, (ed.), Proc. Int. Conf. Pneumoconiosis, Johannesburg, 1969. Oxford University Press, Cape Town, 180.

66. Newhouse, M. L. and Wagner, J. C. (1969). Validation of death certificates in asbestos workers. Brit. J. Indust. Med. 26: 302.

67. Kogan, F. M. Personal communication.

68. Vigliani, E. C. Personal communication.

69. Gilson, J. C. Personal communication.

70. Kiviluoto, R. and Meurman, L. (1970). Results of asbestos exposure in Finland. In: H. A. Shapiro, (ed.), Proc. Int. Conf. Pneumoconiosis, Johannesburg, 1969. Oxford University Press, Cape Town, 190.

71. Hourihane, D. O'B. (1964). The pathology of mesotheliomata and an analysis of their association with asbestos exposure. Thorax 19: 268.

72. Hagerstrand, I., Meurman, L. and Odlund, B. (1968). Asbestos bodies in lungs and mesothelioma. A retrospective examination of a ten-year autopsy material. Acta. Pathol. Microbiol. Scand. 72: 177.

73. Ashcroft, T. and Heppleston, A. G. (1970). Mesothelioma and asbestos on Tyneside. In: H. A. Shapiro, (ed.), Proc. of Int. Conf. Pneumoconiosis, Johannesburg, 1969. Oxford University Press, Cape Town, 177.

PART IV

SOME GENERAL CONSIDERATIONS

CHAPTER 13. IMPLICATIONS OF MULTIPLE FACTORS FOR PREVENTION AND CONTROL

LESTER BRESLOW, School of Public Health,
University of California at Los Angeles

SELECTING ENVIRONMENTAL FACTORS FOR DISEASE CONTROL

In seeking to establish control over disease conditions it is first necessary to take account of all means that may be useful. Such means include education and medical care, as well as environmental measures. A strategy for health improvement must incorporate all three of these approaches which constitute the trimvirate of disease control. Tactical decisions are then necessary from time to time as to which specific measures offer greatest promise.

The strategy of disease control can be illustrated by taking the problem of mortality and morbidity caused by automobile accidents as an example:

CONSIDERATIONS IN CONTROL OF MORTALITY AND MORBIDITY CAUSED BY AUTOMOBILE ACCIDENTS

Environmental Measures	Educational Measures	Medical Care
Construction of streets and highways.	Driver training in vehicle manipulation.	Ambulance and first aid service.
Design and construction of automobiles.	Avoidance of alcohol and other drugs before driving.	Emergency medical service.

Continued on next page.

Environmental Measures	Educational Measures	Medical Care
Road signs and obstacles a) Regular b) Special circumstances (such as repair).	Avoidance of driving during adverse physio-logical states, e.g. fatigue.	Definitive medical care and rehabili-tation.

A comprehensive strategy for controlling mortality and morbidity resulting from automobile accidents (or any other morbid condition) must thus embrace not only the multiple environmental factors that may be involved, but the other major means of disease control, namely, education and medical care.

Assuming that a comprehensive strategy can be laid out, as in the case of automobile injuries, what criteria should be adopted in determining tactics, i.e. in selecting particular control measures for emphasis? While essentially the same criteria can be applied to the selection of educational and medical care as well as environmental measures, we shall consider here mainly the latter type.

An obvious first criterion in the selection process is the relative importance of the factor to be controlled, i. e. the extent to which the particular factor is responsible for the condition under consideration. Given a particular set of road conditions, and certain automobiles exposed to these conditions, is it the condition of the roads or the construction of the automobiles that contributes more to the "accidental" trauma that is to be reduced? The answer to such questions indicates where the emphasis in control efforts should go. While "everything possible should be done", priorities in action must often be established. To take another example, should one concentrate on cigarette smoking or asbestos exposure to control lung cancer? Here again the proportion of disease caused by the particular factors can usually be best established by epidemiological studies.

206

A second consideration is the technical feasibility of control. Returning to the automobile accident example, is it technically more feasible to build safety features into the vehicle or into the road? Whether the means of control, for the one or the other, are in hand or readily attainable would influence the tactical decision.

One would also choose among environmental factors for control at least to some extent on the basis of cost. An inexpensive measure would be preferred, other things being equal, to a costly one. In this connection it is important not to sacrifice a substantial health interest to economic considerations. One can, however, estimate how to achieve a given health objective in the most economical way.

Further, the choice of environmental factor for control should reflect one's expectation as to promptness and effectiveness of the action. In the example given, which can be accomplished more expeditiously, improvement of automobiles on the road or improvement of the roads themselves? How many years would it take to make significant improvement in (a) roads, (b) automobiles; and relatively how effective would each be?

The several criteria mentioned above can be useful guides to selection among multiple environmental factors for control. Decisions about control measures are often made with such criteria vaguely but not systematically in mind. It may be helpful to make them explicit.

Epidemiological studies can be helpful in applying these criteria, especially to the extent that such investigations proceed beyond observation and extend into the experimental realm. Often only trials of actual intervention will elucidate the courses of action to be preferred. In this connection sequential analysis is proving a more and more useful tool, indicating when to proceed with and when to stop alternative methods of intervention.

It is perhaps appropriate here to note another aspect of decision-making about environmental control measures, namely the kind of situation in which a

single environmental condition is involved in several
different disease conditions. The same chemical may
induce carcinogenesis and teratogenesis; cigarette
smoking has been implicated in lung cancer,
bronchitis-emphysema, and myocardial infarction.
Control of certain environmental situations thus may
be important not just for one condition but for
several.

In evaluating the effects of environmental
measures for disease control, it is necessary to
consider the lag in reducing both immediate and
long-term effects. Children with lead poisoning from
ingestion of lead-containing paints, for example, may
still be affected by behavior disorders long after
removal of the paint that is responsible.

INTERRELATIONSHIP OF ENVIRONMENTAL AND
ENDOGENOUS FACTORS

Because of the often complex causation process
which must be dealt with, it should be noted, the
selection and use of environmental control measures
must take into account the possibility of endogenous
factors.

What should be considered endogenous and what
exogenous (environmental) in disease causation is by
no means clear-cut. If environment is defined
broadly enough to include the uterine environment and
previous exposure of genetic material to
environmental factors, it can be said that all
disease is causally related to environmental factors.

To illustrate a common relationship between
environmental and endogenous factors in disease, one
may consider the role of physiologic factors in the
respiratory system in responding to irritant gases
and particles in the respired air. A partial list of
these factors would include the components of the
clearance systems -- the respiratory cilia, mucous
blanket and alveolar macrophages, as well as surface
active agents, immunologic behavior, bronchospasm,
and reflexes. These mechanisms can and do respond in
different ways to ambient mixtures of gases and
particles. The effects may alter responses to
subsequent exposures, as might occur when ciliary
activity is inhibited by sulfur dioxide, with

resulting slowing of clearance of smoke particles, or when nitrogen dioxide diminishes resistance to invasion by micro-organisms. These effects exemplify the interrelatedness of factors in the etiology of disease.

Host resistance to the parasites of malaria may be affected by the presence of other anemia-inducing parasites. Efforts to control the conditions caused by malaria infection should thus take into account intestinal and other parasitic infestation that may be present. Otherwise the anticipated gain in health may not be realized.

When concern about health effects of air pollution began to rise in the 1950's, it was noted that the death rate from pulmonary emphysema was increasing steadily in the United States. The hypothesis that this increase was causally related to community air pollution has still not been proven or disproven. British investigations at about the same time focussed on a chronic nonspecific respiratory disease that was a leading cause of death in the United Kingdom. The manifestations of the disease in Britain were different from what was probably a closely related disease in North America, but studies were easier in Britain because the prevalence of the disease there was far greater than in the United States. This family of chronic nonspecific respiratory diseases turned out to be primarily an affliction of males aged thirty and above, with a very strong social class gradient to the disadvantage of the lowest social classes. At least three groups of factors were clearly involved: an effect of age which might include physiologic or constitutional factors, or length of exposure, or both; an effect of sex which also could represent physiologic differences or a sex-associated difference of exposure; and finally a group of influences that are often grouped under the heading of socio-economic factors.

As studies progressed it became clear that cigarette smoking was so closely associated with chronic respiratory disease that smoking habits had to be known before other risks could be evaluated. Another very important factor which has hitherto been too little appreciated in the U. S. is the association of various kinds of occupational exposure with specific or nonspecific chronic respiratory diseases. Much of the sex difference in incidence and prevalence of these diseases is accounted for by the sex difference in smoking habits and in occupational exposures. Although the kinds of respiratory exposure can be separated in a broad sense, each one in fact is a complex mixture of gases and fine particulates, usually of poorly defined composition and character. Biologic effects can be due to individual components or to the product of intereactions between them; the results may be additive or synergistic. An example of the latter is the apparently greater risk in cigarette smokers of developing lung cancer after exposure to asbestos fibers or to radium daughter products in uranium mines. (See Chapter 5).

Another major cause of death which has been increasing in frequency in the U. S. in recent years is cirrhosis of the liver. Looked at broadly from an environmental point of view, there are several similarities between this disease and chronic nonspecific respiratory disease. In the U. S. the age distributions are about the same, the male sex is most afflicted, and there is the same kind of social class gradient, with the lowest classes having the highest incidence of cirrhosis. As in the case of the respiratory disease etiology, the primary cause of cirrhosis is a personal habit -- the consumption of alcoholic beverages, presumably in excessive amounts. Other major factors suspected of playing a role in causation are nutritional deficiencies, viral hepatitis, and hepatotoxic chemicals other than alcohol. Each of these factors under experimental circumstances is capable of being a primary cause of cirrhosis, but in real life they frequently occur together, especially in the case of alcohol and nutritional deficiency. The extent to which these factors may be additive or synergistic in man has not been thoroughly explored. Known interactions support the concept of universality of multifactor causation of malfunction or disease. (See Chapter 3).

For example, alcohol ingestion increases susceptibility to damage from halogenated hydrocarbon solvents. Ethyl alcohol is one of a large number of chemicals found capable of inducing liver microsomal enzymes. Since the chemicals that can induce or

210

inhibit microsomal enzymes include commonly used drugs such as phenobarbital and ubiquitous environmental pollutants such as DDT, it is desirable to learn how significant these interactions are at exposure levels which occur in specific population groups. Determining the exposure history of liver cells will be even more difficult than quantifying the exposure history of lungs. Considering the central role of the liver in metabolic transformations of drugs and environmental chemicals, one might be concerned about specific associations of occupational exposures with cirrhosis or even with hepatic cancer. The frequency of cirrhosis does vary with occupation but not in a way that clearly links the disease with industrial exposure. (See Chapters 7, 8, 9).

Thus the decisions about environmental control measures should be taken in the light of all available knowledge of endogenous as well as environmental factors in the causation-pathogenesis process.

ENVIRONMENTAL AND HUMAN SURVEILLANCE AS THE BASIS FOR PLANNING CONTROL MEASURES

Technological advances are bringing larger and larger population groups under exposure to hazardous chemical and physical conditions. No longer are such exposures limited to small groups of individuals who are in reasonably good health and employed in certain industrial situations. New products that are widely used and new environmental conditions, such as air pollution, affect virtually the entire population.

This means that protective measures must incorporate consideration for the most sensitive individuals of a population -- the very young, the elderly, the feeble as well as the robust -- those whose endogenous state may make them highly vulnerable to conditions that do not cause any damage to the vast majority. For example, infirm and aged persons in nursing homes suffer a sharply increased mortality rate when the temperature rises from a daily high of 80-85° F. to more than 100° F. for a few days. Mortality among these same infirm and aged persons does not seem to increase with the intensity of photochemical smog, but the level of smog does affect respiratory function in persons already suffering from severe respiratory impairment.

Routine surveillance of water (for bacterial content and chlorine residual) and of milk (for bacteria and evidence of pasteurization), coupled with reporting and investigation of bacterial diseases in the population using the water and milk, has been the hallmark of control over those diseases. Now we have entered an era with a different constellation of environmental hazards and diseases. It will be necessary to maintain a wide surveillance network covering physical and chemical factors in the environment that may cause damage to human function, as well as those human functions themselves that may be adversely affected.

Monitoring broad trends in general health (amount of disability, anxiety, and the like, as in the U. S. National Health Survey) is desirable as one basis for considering possible environmental relationships. Also, of course, specific health conditions should be monitored in connection with more specific environmental situations suspected of being causative; for example; mesothelioma of the lung for its relationship to asbestos exposure, and hearing loss for its relationship to the noise level in cities.

Comparable monitoring of environmental hazards, such as crowding (for its possible effect on general health), asbestos exposure, and noise should be undertaken.

Just as monitoring both typhoid fever in a community and the bacterial quality of the community water supply were helpful in reducing an environmentally caused disease, it is to be anticipated that monitoring both hearing loss and noise-levels will prove useful in reducing another environmentally caused condition. The rise of the decibel level in cities is an increasingly important factor causing damage to human function. Not only does it result in distraction and other possible harm at the time of noise, but continued over long periods the latter can result in serious hearing loss. The steadily mounting decibel level in cities illustrates well the need for a preventive approach to environmental health problems based on surveillance. Shall cities delay action against noise until it causes permanent hearing loss to substantial numbers of persons?

One essential element, therefore, in control of environmentally induced disease is a surveillance system that monitors both the chemical, physical, and other aspects of the environment which are suspected of causing disease, and the human functions that may be affected. Some experience has already been gained with this kind of surveillance in monitoring: carbon monoxide, sulfur dioxide, oxidants, lead, radioactivity, particulate matter and other possible adverse factors in air pollution; and certain symptoms in the general population, deaths of infirm persons, and lead storage in highly exposed groups which might be related to air pollutants.

The surveillance system should include, and in fact emphasize, data linking environmental conditions with their health effects. For example, systematic studies of mortality and morbidity on the one hand and occupations on the other have yielded many important clues concerning the environmental origin of disease. Investigations of adverse drug reactions also illustrate the value of more systematic attention to possible linkages between disease conditions and the environment.

The rapidity of technological advances, the extent of environmental changes that have already occurred, and the often long latent period before adverse human effects become obvious (and can be corrected) require serious and immediate attention to this matter of environmental and human surveillance for detection of situations requiring control.

IMPLEMENTATION OF CONTROL MEASURES

After identification of environmental factors in disease that should be controlled, the first issue usually arising is the feasibility of control measures. Whether it be automobile exhaust control, avoidance of stream pollution or location of nuclear power plants, those motivated by the economic benefit of avoiding control react initially by denying any hazard, and then by pointing the finger at some other source of the environmental factor. When it is settled that a hazard in fact exists, and that it arises at least in substantial part from a particular source, the question of feasibility of control measures is next.

Exploration of this problem quickly exposes its two aspects: (1) technical, and (2) economic. The technical means for controlling the environmental factor may first have to be developed and tested; thereafter the amount and allocation of cost must be faced. Resolving the many issues that arise in determining the technical and economic feasibility of environmental control measures, especially when their resolution is costly, involves a mixture (one might say a maelstrom) of science and technology, public education, and economic forces expressed politically.

The existence of multiple factors and multiple sources of the same factor (for example, carbon monoxide from cigarette smoke, automobile exhaust, and stationary sources) makes control all the more formidable. The complexity of a particular situation often makes it extremely difficult to array the several possible control measures for serious consideration in the light of the criteria cited earlier. For example, it may be more effective and even less expensive to build more bedrooms for the control of respiratory-spread diseases in general than to attack these diseases one by one on more specific bases. Yet such an issue rarely even comes to attention.

Multiple environmental factors may interact in quite unexpected ways, complicating approaches to control. Thus two classes of pesticides, EPN and malathion, were found to potentiate one another. This effect which persists for about 12 days after exposure has still not been used as a basis for setting exposure standards. Scientific understanding requires consideration of many variables, public education becomes a more complex task since no single thing is culpable, and those resisting change find it easier to confound and delay the necessary economic and political decisions. (See Chapter 7).

In such a situation the most important guide is scientific understanding, of both potential as well as actual hazards to the human condition, and of the technical aspects of control measures. The ultimate decision to act usually comes only when scientists, public educators, and representatives of the political economic power get into the same arena. Effectiveness in that arena is enhanced by understanding the origins, directions, and strengths of these several forces; commitment to one's point of view, even when that is backed by scientific understanding of the environmental problem, is not enough. In the effort to implement control measures scientists must exercise great care in communication with the public, avoiding both understatement and overstatement, and they can be obviously more effective if they understand the economic consequences of control.

HEALTH AS A VALUE IN ENVIRONMENTAL CONTROL

The current world-wide concern about the environment reflects a struggle over fundamental human values.

One aspect of this struggle is the extent to which the individual or the small group can act irrespective of impact on the larger group. At different rates of speed and in various ways throughout the world, that issue is being decided in favor of protecting the larger group.

A more difficult matter is the criteria for determining what is best for the larger group, ultimately society as a whole. Perhaps general agreement could be reached on some such goal as quality of life. Is the latter, however, to be approached on the basis of assuring economic advance, avoiding immediate aesthetic offense, minimizing the possibility of long range damage to health, or on some other basis? Different answers to this question, or at least different emphases, may be given according to one's place in society and the state of social development. Water and air pollution by a factory may be condoned in certain times and places, for example, when economic advance is paramount; but not in others.

Those communities and nations now undergoing rapid industrial development may wish to profit from the experience of others who have already passed through that phase -- not to hamper industrial development but to avoid its undesirable and unnecessary side-effects. It is clear in retrospect that, in the United States and other technologically advanced countries, a large part of the current environmental problem could have been avoided by giving more attention to protection of the environment year by year, and paying for it with each step along the way. Now the economic cost will be huge and the present generation at least suffers degradation in the quality of its life. One of the major, current problems in international health is how nations just entering upon industrialization can avoid the tragedies of lung cancer, coronary heart disease and other disease manifestations of life in the so-called advanced countries. Many of these major diseases of our times have resulted from largely unplanned manipulations of the environment that took place without consideration of health consequences.

Sometimes the element of personal choice is advanced as an alternative to environmental control. Although all persons living in certain cities must necessarily breathe polluted air, no one is compelled to use cigarettes, alcohol, or heroin. Involvement with any of the latter obviously depends upon the choices of individuals. Such choices, however, are not "free" in the sense of being uninfluenced by external conditions. The availability and degree of encouragement for an individual to use cigarettes, alcohol, or heroin is clearly subject to social control. The nature and extent of that social control is, in effect, an environmental circumstance profoundly affecting the corresponding adverse health effects that are now so well known. "Personal choice" in such matters, it may truly be said, largely reflects social control.

The broad WHO definition of health -- "physical, mental, and social well-being" -- applied to the current and immediately following generations, may be accepted as the major if not the ultimate criterion of quality of life. If so, then health in this broad sense of well-being should be advanced much more vigorously than heretofore as the basis for environmental decision making. Too often in so-called developed nations throughout the world such decisions are based on narrow, short range economic incentives.

Overcoming this tendency will require a strong commitment to health as a criterion in controlling the multiple factors in the environment that may endanger health. This commitment in a nation may be tested by the extent to which: (1) scientific investigation of the health aspects of the environment is pursued; (2) health protection is the basis for setting standards of environmental quality; (3) emphasis is given to the prevention of possible adverse health effects, not just those confirmed by damage to a whole generation; (4) there is biomedical participation in environmental monitoring; and (5) the planning and operation of environmental control measures are related to a broad strategy for improving the health of the nation, a strategy that correlates health and environmental problem-sheds, and embraces medical, educational, and environmental approaches to health problems.

CHAPTER 14. COMMENTS AND PERSPECTIVES

DOUGLAS H. K. LEE,
National Institute of Environmental Health Sciences,
Research Triangle Park, North Carolina

The field of environmental health is notoriously divided between the enthusiasts who seem to detect a threat in almost all aspects of technological progress, and those who feel that, with a few well publicized exceptions, the world will take care of itself. The narrower question dealt with here -- the extent to which environmental agents must be regarded as operating in complex patterns rather than as independent factors -- shares this polarization.

A special element of conservatism operates here as a legacy from the past. The introduction of the germ theory of disease at the turn of the century shed a brilliant light on the nature and causation of much of the illness then prevalent. Here, at last, was a unifying theory which permitted causes to be sought, prevention to be introduced, and therapy to be prescribed in a systematic manner never before possible. Unfortunately, the bright light concealed as much in its shadows as it revealed in its glare, and non-infectious diseases were relegated to the vague status of diatheses, or simply regarded as breakdowns to be expected in a complex system.

As control of infectious disease progresses, as environmental contaminants increase, and as more is known about pathological responses to contaminants, the true nature of some of these temporarily neglected diseases and dysfunctions has become clearer. Unfortunately, however, the very success of the germ theory encouraged a belief in a simplistic chain of causation -- one specific organism giving rise to one (more or less)

specific disease. It is only with reluctance that
one forsakes the shelter of a simplistic faith to
embrace that of multiple causation. In all
fairness, of course, it must be admitted that a
detailed knowledge of cellular processes, the
primary locus of toxicant effects, is of quite
recent origin, and that mathematical means for
dealing with complexities are still aborning. It was
to stress the complexity of environmental effects
that the topic of multiple factors in the
causation of environmentally related disease was
selected for the fourth book of the Fogarty-NIEHS
series.

As was expected, the contributors' views revealed
the complexity of the problem, and the variety
of attitudes that its complexity permits.
Abundantly clear is the lack of hard data where
they are most needed for appraisal.

Three orders of complexity were discussed:
(a) the multiplicity of environmental agents that can
impinge on the body; (b) the extreme variability in
the reaction of exposed organisms to incident
conditions; and (c) the wide range of
considerations to be evaluated in selecting the
most efficient method of control. Within each
set several subsets were identified. Different
environmental factors may react with one another
to produce new substances that add to
exposure, as is the case with sunlight, ozone, and
hydrocarbon emissions in producing peroxyacetyl
nitrate (PAN). The fate of substances entering the
body is determined, not only by "normal"
pharmacological reactions, but also by the state
of endocrine and other physiological processes
at the time. Public acceptance, economic
feasibility, and efficacy of control measures,
each comprizing many facets, interact to produce
some unexpected and even bizarre reactions to
control measures, as many a would-be reformer has
found to his chagrin.

It is manifestly impossible to deal with all
patterns of all variables; but neither is it possible
to rely solely on information obtained by studying
them one at a time in isolation. Some way must be
taken of selecting those variables, and those
combinations of variables, that offer the greatest

threat to health. This is not an easy task, and the person who makes the selection is going to be called upon repeatedly to justify his choices.

Many bases have been suggested for selection, but three stand out as being particularly important. The most cogent, of course, is the importance of the probable disturbance, having regard to the numbers of people at risk as well as the severity of dysfunction that is produced. But the applicability of this criterion turns on the extent and reliability of the evidence available. In a few instances, like the oft quoted blue cheese episode, we have some firm indications, but in most instances we do not. The defensive phrase, "we have no evidence that these conditions are harmful to man", has no substance if no one has really looked. Epidemiological inquiries could elicit evidence by examination of populations exposed to a particular pattern of environmental factors, but it would first be necessary to establish that it is this pattern, and not some other factor or factors, that is the operating determinant. To a certain extent this smacks of proceeding in a circle; it is likely to be effective only in reinforcing a prima facie case that has been established by some other means. It is ironic that it sometimes appears easier to make a case for controlling a single agent that is only part of the threat, than it is for dealing with an interactive group of factors that is the real offender.

A second basis for selection is argument by analogy. If certain chemicals, acting on individuals under certain physiological conditions, are known to produce an adverse effect, then chemicals of similar structure and properties, acting under similar conditions, are likely to produce corresponding effects. This line of reasoning has more chance of being successful if the mechanisms by which the effects are produced (e.g., transformation by hepatic microsomes) are known. Considerable use has been made in this connection of information gained in the study of therapeutic drugs, as is evident in several of the preceding contributions. Animal experimentation, of course, can be a powerful tool in establishing mechanisms and the probability of adverse effects from new patterns of exposure; but there is always the final question as to how far animal experimentation indicates the threat that the same exposure would pose for man. Techniques for extrapolation are improving, but the question has to be faced.

A third criterion that has to be taken into account is the frequency with which the adverse pattern in question can be expected to occur. This, in turn, leads to some "sticky" questions, such as whether a severe effect occurring only occasionally or a lesser effect happening frequently should receive prior attention. The cognate question, as to how much risk can be accepted, is one that administrators must face, but with understandable reluctance. When the question is rephrased with an economic element included -- how much risk is needed to justify the economic disturbance produced by control? -- the going gets stickier than ever. Unfortunately for the investigating scientist, these questions cannot be postponed to some indefinite future; they affect his choice of which pattern of multiple factors out of an infinite range should be selected for study.

If we turn from consideration of specific environmental agents to the other end of the spectrum, disease states which may owe their development at least in part to environmental causes, the area of uncertainty increases. While it is true that the environmental origins of some diseases, such as cancer, are now well established, there are other diseases for which current explanations are inadequate. Putting aside for the moment conditions attributable to genetic defects or to aging (in which environmental factors may still be involved in secondary fashion), there remain a number of disturbances for which a satisfying explanation has not been established. Smoking and respiratory infection certainly affect the symptoms of a person with emphysema, for example, but it is not clear what are original causes of the condition. It is tempting to think that various environmental insults, operating over a lifetime prolonged by protection from acute infectious disease, are responsible for such a condition; but hard proof is lacking. It is very difficult in a patient of 50 to determine what environmental insult may have started him on the emphysematous path at the age of 10. The increasing prevalence of emphysema indicates the need for identifying and controlling the cause or causes. The environmental health scientist may believe that the causative factors are multiple, with different combinations operating in different persons. Hopes that a reduction of urban air pollution will automatically bring about a diminution of the causative factors are simply hopes. We are not yet in a position to say that any set of pollutants in particular really causes the condition, or even that the cause is actually a pollutant.

The intellectual problem of handling several factors of varying intensity and effect is formidable. It is one thing to discuss the importance of multiple factor recognition in qualitative terms as has been done in previous chapters; but the actual handling and interpretation of hard data is fraught with difficulties. Some helpful mathematical techniques are developing, however. For nearly two decades certain methods of fitting response surfaces to biological data have been used in agricultural and industrial chemical problem analysis, but have been largely neglected in pharmacological and toxicological studies. While these are most easily applied for relatively simple linear functions, they can also be adapted to non-linear functions. In parallel fashion, mathematical modelling of biological systems involving several factors, using difference and differential equations, find increasing use in problems of energy transfer. It would seem, also, that the iterative processes used to bring lunar terrain features into prominence against background noise could be adapted to revealing significant events in a mass of environmental response data. Marine ecologists are utilizing some of these methods; it would seem profitable for the toxicologist to meet the mathematicians part way.

The role of the clinician in treating persons inflicted with chronic diseases, and particularly those of environmental origin, is a difficult one, somewhat removed from the classical concept of a successful healer. To the extent that the pathological changes in these patients are irreversible, which is usually the case, his preoccupation will be with conservation of existing function rather than the effecting of a cure. To the extent that the basic causes are buried in the irretrievable past, and particularly where the pattern varies with the individual, he may well feel that a precise definition of etiology, on which disease classification tends to be based, is not necessary, or even possible. (Under existing compensation laws and practices, of course, the fixation of "blame" for a person's disease assumes large legal importance, and its establishment will continue to plague all concerned).

Concern about future attitudes in this increasingly uncertain situation affects more than the physician. All those who deal with environmental impacts on health, from the laboratory scientist, through control authorities, to the industrial producer and the individual consumer have cause to be concerned. Clearly we cannot continue to deal in simplistic fashion with affairs that are very complex. Somehow we must learn to recognize what combinations are most important, and try to deal with them. This in turn calls for greater acceptance by regulators that the obvious and direct approach may not always be successful, and that careful thought needs to be given to possible repercussions of a biological as well as of an economic nature. Since no amount of foresight is going to reveal all of the possibilities, a constant state of inquiry and alertness for new situations must be maintained. Needed above all is intimate and continuous communication between the investigative scientist and the regulator, whereby the possibilities are constantly presented to the latter, and leads provided to the former. Inasmuch as a fourth set of complexities, not discussed in this volume -- complexities in the regulatory machinery -- is inherent in today's civilization, communication of information and coordination of action are far from simple and automatic. However comprehensive and sophisticated electronic communication becomes, its effective use will continue to depend upon human motivation -- motivation by the investigator to make his findings readily available, and motivation by the controller to make himself aware of the information, even if it makes his decision process more difficult. There will be difficulties and resistances, but a workable conspectus will eventually develop; one hopes that this will come to pass before too many beguiling paths have been followed to an unprofitable end.